RELIEVE
MENSTRUAL PAIN
WITH HERBAL REMEDIES

ANCESTRAL HEALING
KNOWLEDGE OF WOMEN

Practical guide

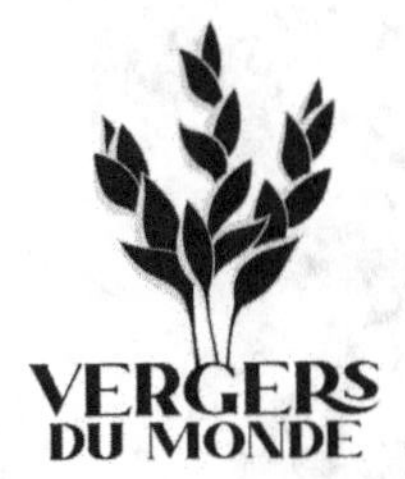

Women are the living libraries of traditions,
carrying within them the stories of the past and the
hopes of the future.

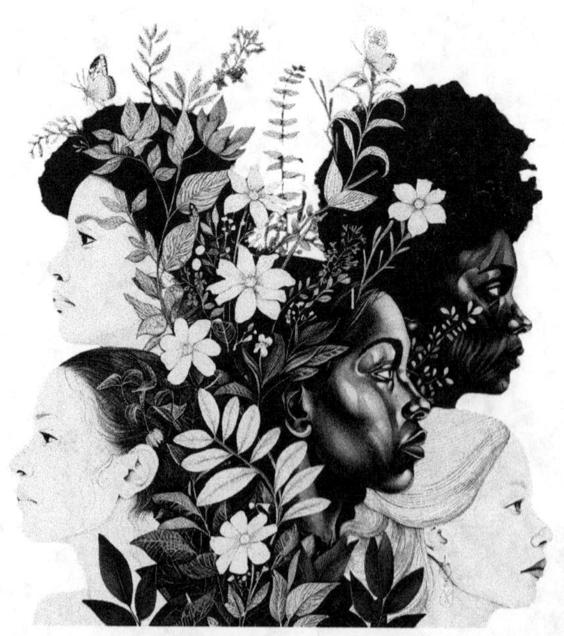

Summary

ABOUT VERGERS DU MONDE

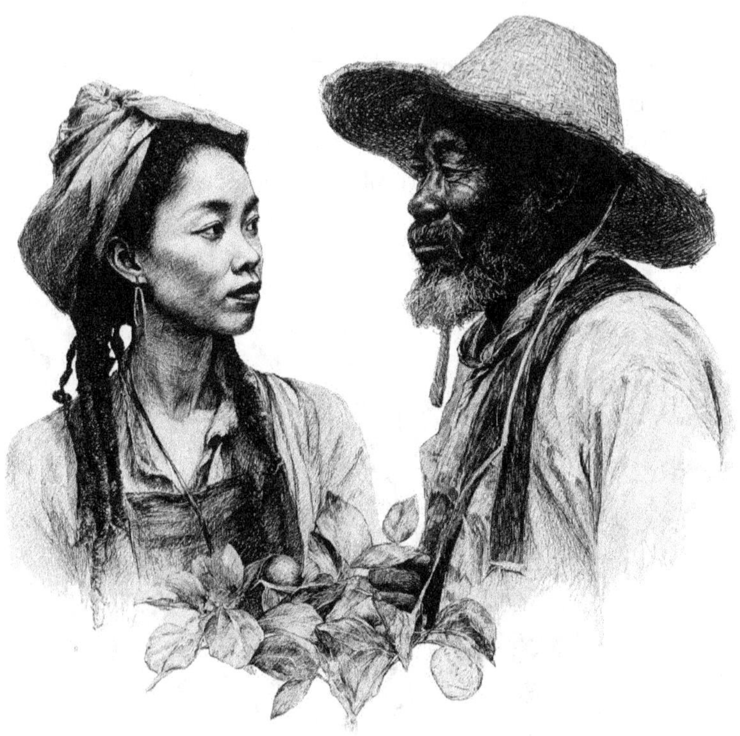

At Vergers du Monde, we walk beside those who cultivate the earth. Farmers and herders, wherever they come from, carry within them knowledges shaped by patience, observation, and dialogue with living landscapes. Our work begins there: in the encounter, in the field visit, in the workshop where gestures are exchanged and words take root.

We see these practices as part of an intangible human heritage, one that deserves recognition and transmission. Our role is not to reshape or appropriate these knowledges, but to serve as a resonator, to amplify the voices of farming communities, to highlight their contexts, and to ensure their contributions are heard and respected. We believe that this knowledge is not only about the past: it is one of our strongest chances to hold steady and live in harmony on this earth.

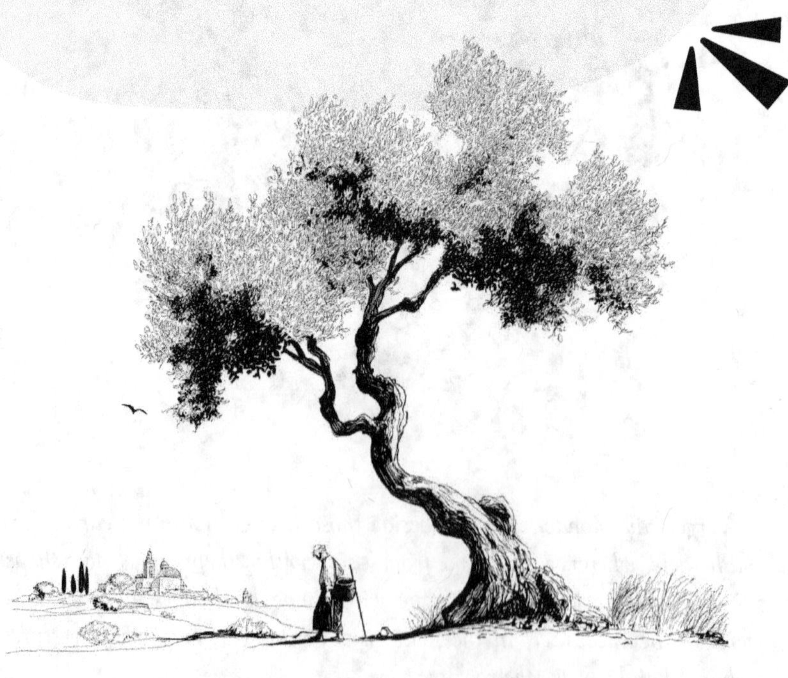

CULTIVATE YOUR TRADITIONAL ECOLOGICAL KNOWLEDGE

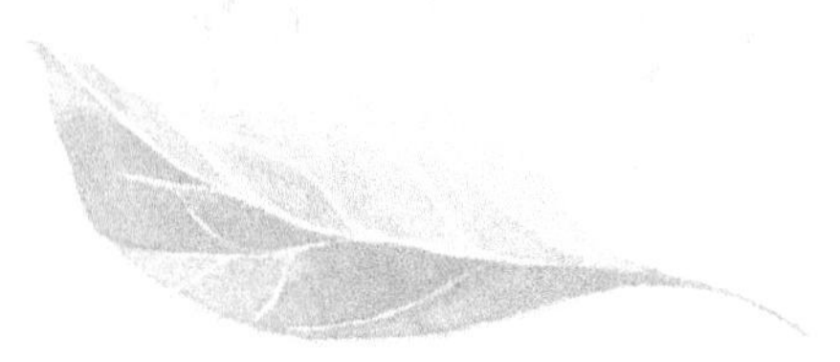

This is what we call Traditional Ecological Knowledge (TEK): a body of wisdom shaped by generations of cultivators around the globe. The expression itself was brought into use in the 1980s within academic circles, as a way to affirm that such knowledge deserved to stand alongside scientific methods in conservation and environmental thinking. Since then, much has been written about how to frame different knowledge systems. But for us, the essential point is simple: TEK has too often been pushed aside, when in fact it remains indispensable.

TEK lives in crop rotations that protect fertility, in water-saving techniques that anticipate scarcity, in the stewardship of seeds, and in the quiet art of reading seasons, skies, and soils. It travels through stories, shared work, and the attentive practice of farming. And it is not static: it adapts constantly to new lands, new climates, and new challenges.

Restoring TEK to its rightful place does not mean setting it against science. It means allowing both to enrich each other, science offering models and analysis, TEK grounding us in lived practice and resilience.

This book continues that work. It seeks to honor TEK not as a resource to be extracted, but as a living heritage to be respected in the voices of the communities that carry it, because their wisdom is also our path to a sustainable and balanced future.

FOREWORD

Please be aware that this manual does not offer medical guidance or therapy and does not purport to replace expert advice. Our aim is to expand your perspectives by acquainting you with traditional techniques from different cultures and periods, enabling individuals to extract what resonates with them. This endeavor contributes to the advancement of ancestral wisdom and an ethnographic investigation into the understanding and customs linked to the utilization and alteration of flora worldwide, rather than a medical standpoint. Should a health concern arise, we advise you to seek guidance from a healthcare professional.

FOR WHOM IS THIS PRACTICAL GUIDE INTENDED?

Do you experience intense menstrual discomfort like severe cramps, endometriosis, or other menstrual cycle-related conditions? Have you ever wondered how women worldwide have turned to plants for centuries to ease their suffering? Are you seeking practical guidance, a life philosophy, or natural solutions to enhance your comprehension and handling of your physical well-being?

You have arrived at the perfect destination.

Embark on a captivating exploration through the medicinal legacies of women worldwide. Travel from Africa to Asia, across the Americas and Europe, unveiling ancient traditions, botanical wonders, time-honored cures, and nurturing ceremonies passed down through generations. Immerse yourself in this rich tapestry of heritage and unearth the wisdom to alleviate your suffering naturally and holistically.

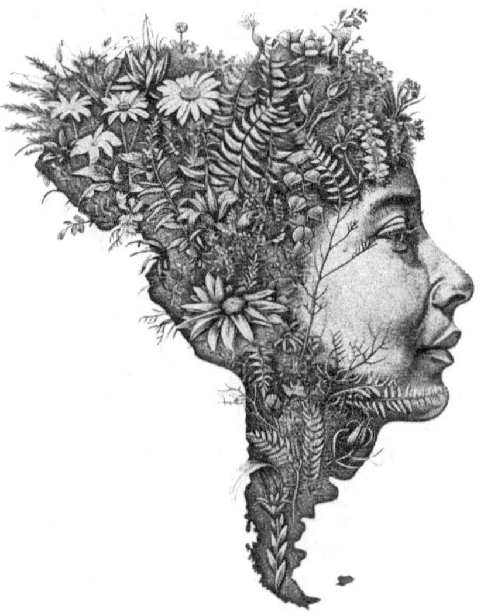

Uphold and Acknowledge

In a world of constant change, where traditions may be at risk of fading, it is vital to safeguard the ancient wisdom that forms the essence of local communities. This wisdom, passed down through generations, is not merely cultural heritage; it embodies a profound bond with nature and a diligently acquired insight.

The secrecy encompassing these rituals is crucial to safeguard their essence. We dedicate ourselves to recording this wisdom with profound reverence, seeking the approval of those who impart it and recognizing its source. Every plant, every ceremony, every cure is grounded in a particular heritage that merits acknowledgment in its entirety and variety.

It is crucial to recall that these customs form a vital aspect of the cultural and spiritual essence of the communities that originated them. They are frequently passed down subtly, within the confines of privacy, and it is this very subtlety that safeguards their significance and worth. By honoring these practices, we play a part in conserving a priceless legacy, all the while acknowledging the sagacity and strength of the women who persist in upholding them.

Women embody the essence of medicinal plant wisdom. Throughout history, from ancient midwives to modern herbalists, our bond with plants and their transformative abilities endures as powerful and essential.

ROSE, J. (2001). 375 ESSENTIAL OILS AND HYDROSOLS. FROG, LTD.

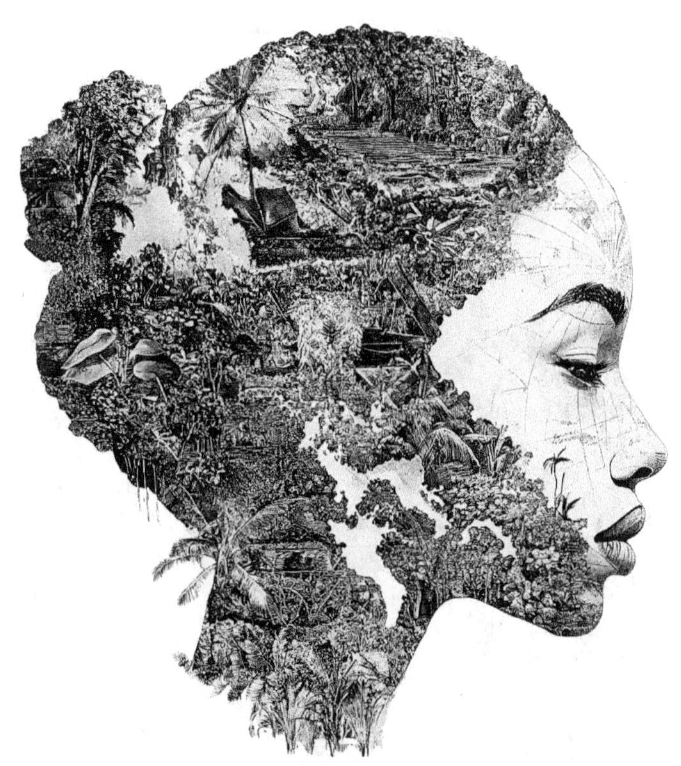

METHODOLOGY

To create this transformative manual, Vergers du Monde embraced a captivating and enlightening method, intertwining personal narratives, group dialogues, and thorough investigation.

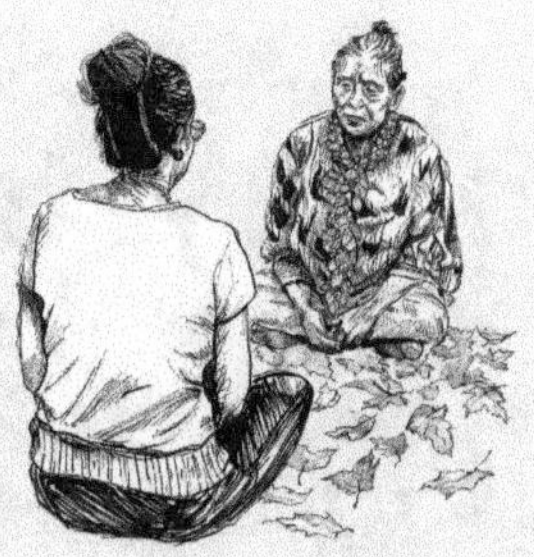

We embarked on a journey of meaningful one-on-one conversations with women from various backgrounds. Facilitated by a knowledgeable social science researcher, these interactions unveiled personal narratives and distinct practices of utilizing plants for alleviating menstrual discomfort. Every discussion unveiled valuable insights into traditional wisdom and captivating cultural intricacies, providing a profound and vibrant outlook.

To enhance these accounts, Vergers du Monde orchestrated group sessions uniting women from diverse backgrounds, whether French or from other places. These sessions served as genuine meeting points for sharing, where the participants openly traded their expertise and methods regarding medicinal plants. These exchanges not only enriched our guide with numerous viewpoints but also fostered deep connections and promoted the passing on of wisdom across generations.

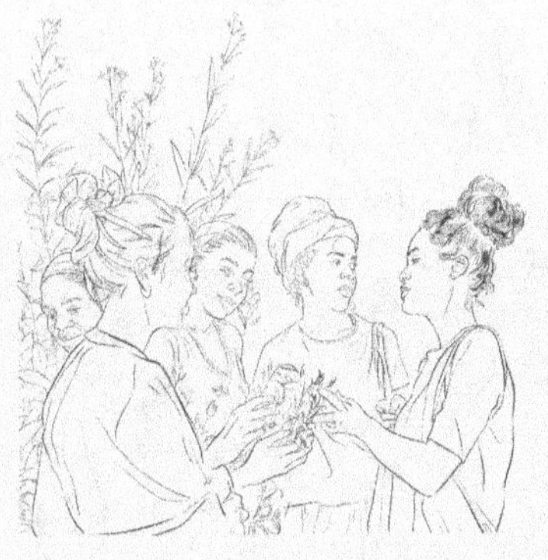

Finally, immersing into a sea of documentary exploration has not only contextualized but also enriched the gathered information. Vergers du Monde delved into academic, ethnobotanical, and historical references to guarantee the precision and significance of the featured remedies. This meticulous and fervent method secures that the manual is rooted in sturdy grounds, thereby providing genuine and trustworthy guidance, all the while championing age-old customs across the globe.

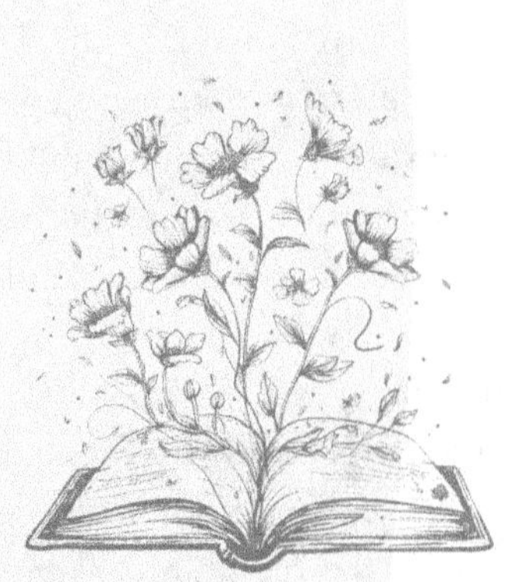

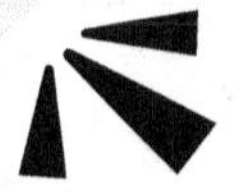

In the West, reflecting on our history

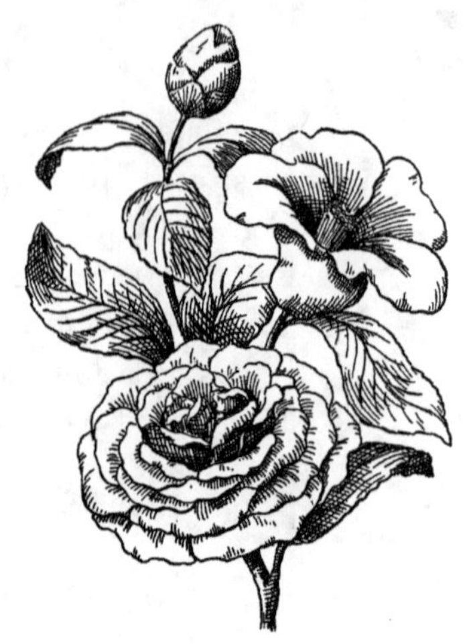

For years, our team have explored farms in France and worldwide, guided by the tales of migrant farmers. Our journey led us to uncover an agriculture predominantly characterized by mechanization and groundbreaking innovations. Within this contemporary setting, we observed women often being marginalized. Despite their pivotal roles during the World Wars in Europe, stepping in for men on the front lines, women continued to be steadfast pillars of agriculture, albeit unseen. In France, prior to 1980, the official recognition of a farmer's spouse was nonexistent, despite rural women significantly contributing to agricultural and household duties.

In the West, what then of the knowledge held by women? Have they been forgotten with the wheat under the combine harvester, or have they been persevered through what we now refer to as grandmother's remedies. We will seek to address this by taking a comparative perspective, examining the wealth of wisdom and traditions across the globe.

Wisdom in isolation

At the same time, another narrative unfolds. Remaining in France, we encounter Aissata, Dania, Nour, Maria, Ling, and Elira. Their tales differ, yet they share two common threads: the necessity to depart their homelands, each for unique reasons. From Albania, Mauritania, China, Tunisia, Mexico, or Syria, each one carries the wisdom of their ancestors, a heritage transmitted through the ages, from mother to daughter. Some departed from rural lands where farming sustained their families. Let's delve deeper into traditional farming, into the land, for this wisdom is deeply intertwined with a specific time and place.

A woman's touch holds more precision than a man's.

Some of these women in exile hail from communities where they fulfill a tangible function as cultivators, collaborating in field duties alongside men. For instance, Tenzin, a Tibetan farmer, shared with us in an interview that during planting seasons, a woman's touch is often more precise than a man's, their movements naturally harmonizing with each other.

In every community, women hold profound wisdom about plants, not just for nourishment but also for healing.

In the realm of healing, consider the Fulani people of the Sahel. Here, women embody the essence of traditional healers, utilizing herbal remedies to address a myriad of ailments. Rooted in wisdom cascading through time, these practices underscore the significance of preserving ancestral knowledge within the fabric of community well-being and heritage.

It proved to be a challenging task for us to condense this valuable wisdom into one cohesive piece. We organized it by geographical era, continent by continent, blending testimonies and traditions from all around the globe. We encourage you to explore these diverse cultures, each contributing its distinct wealth. By sharing the gathered stories, our aim is to present a glimpse of the beauty and variety of women's plant knowledge.

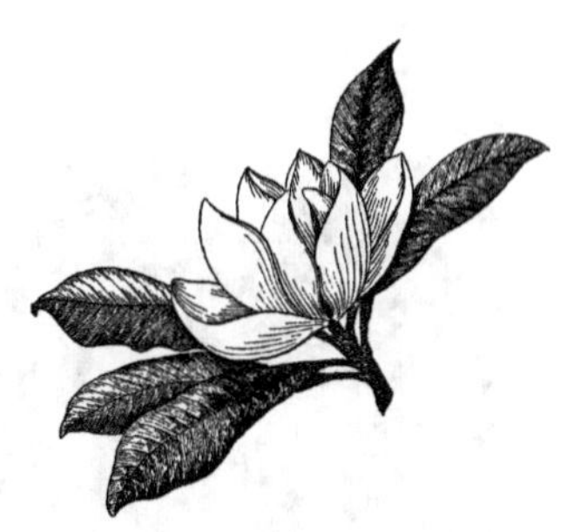

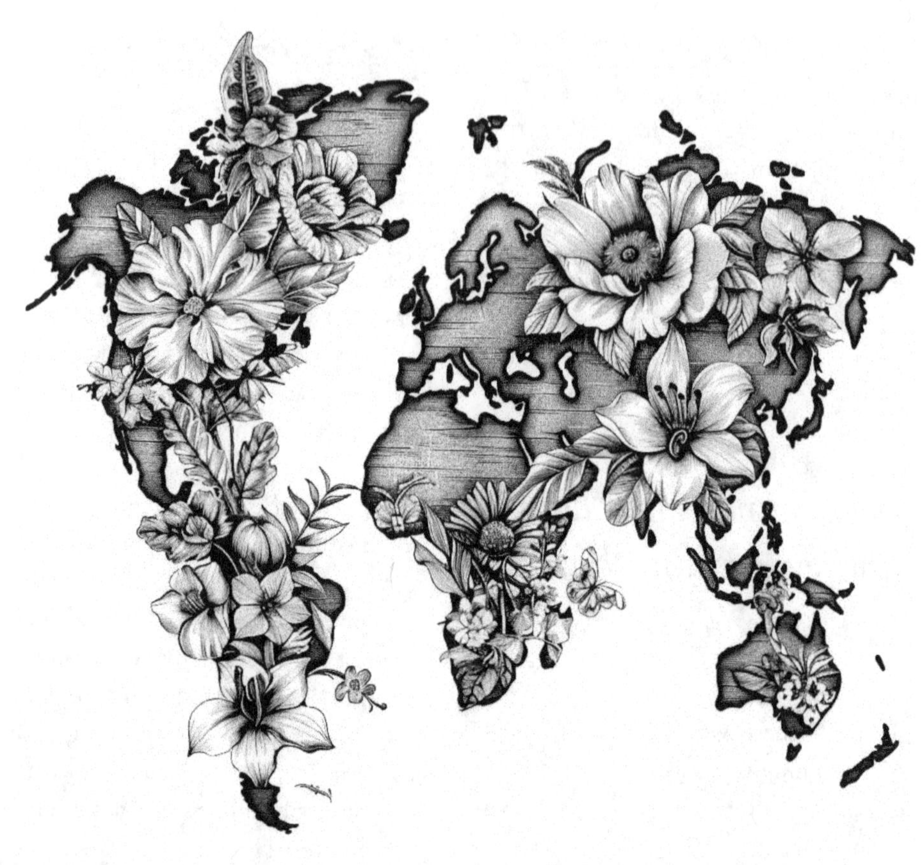

EMBARK ON YOUR
GLOBAL JOURNEY NOW.

CHAPTER 1
Africa

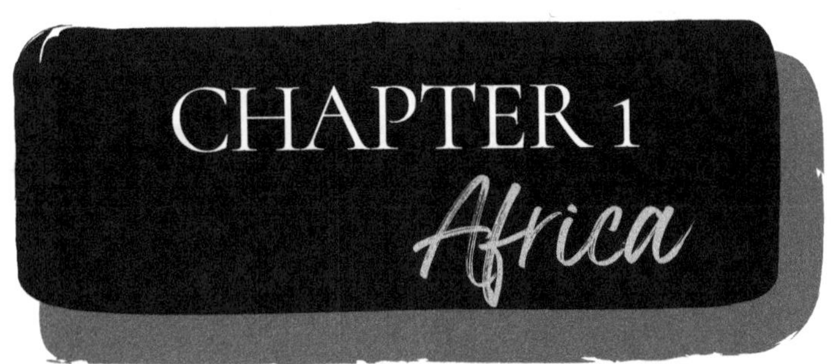

SENEGAL REGION RIVER

NORTH AFRICA

GREAT LAKES REGION

INDIAN OCEAN ISLANDS

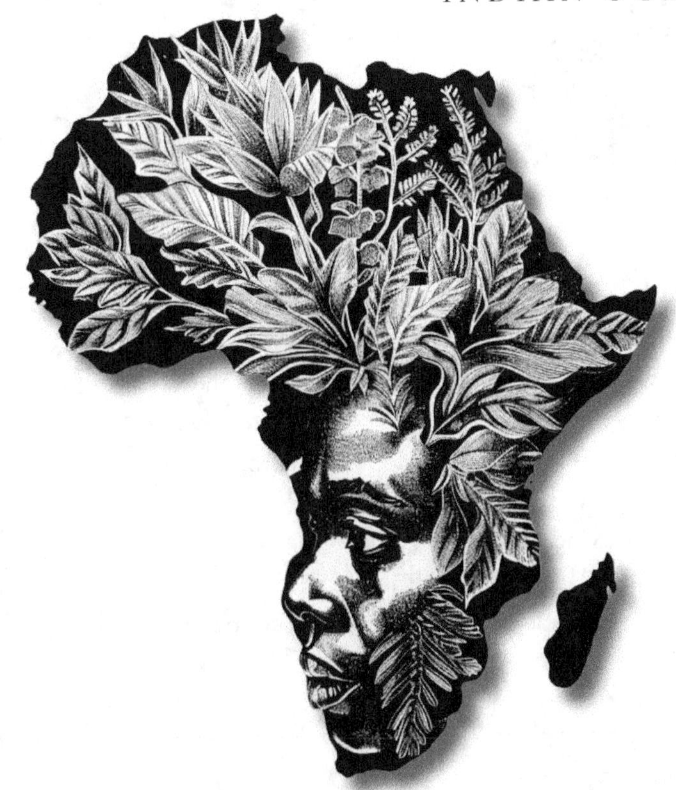

Senegal Region River

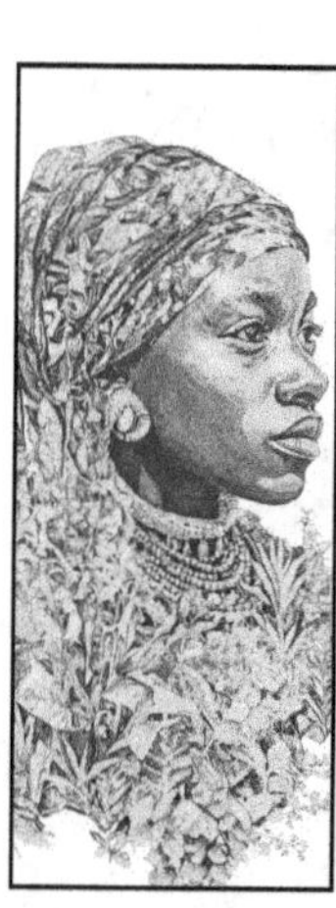
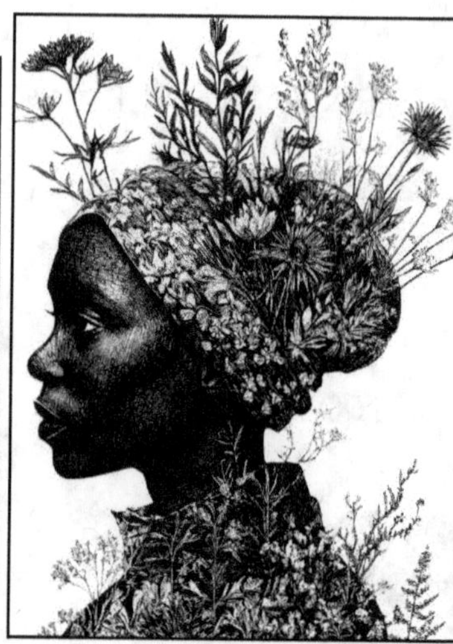
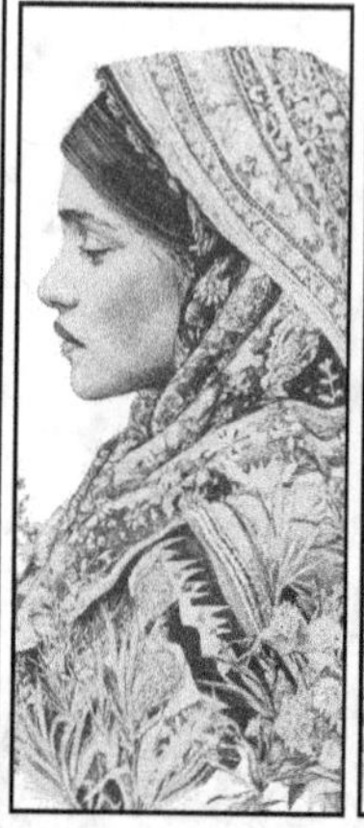
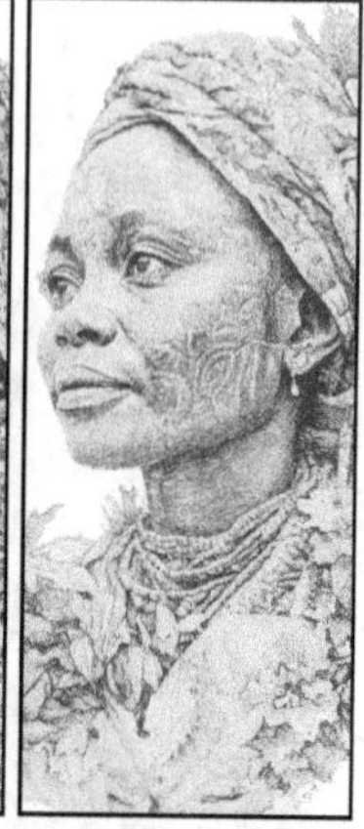

Embark on a remarkable journey tracing the path of the Senegal River, a significant waterway in West Africa. Originating from the Fouta Djalon Mountains in Guinea, it meanders through various nations such as Senegal, Mauritania, and Mali, before gracefully merging with the vast Atlantic Ocean.

This expedition is a testament to the beauty and power of nature. Fertile lands, once the cradle of ancient civilizations like the kingdom of Tekrour, still hold a vital position in the region's agriculture. They are rich in traditional wisdom, not just in farming techniques but also in the healing properties of plants.

Traditions

The essence of traditional medicine in West Africa lies in the wisdom passed down through generations. This wisdom is safeguarded by select groups of initiated individuals, including traditional healers and herbalists (Gueye, 2019). In nations like Senegal, Mali, and Mauritania, these customs are intricately woven into local traditions and convictions, forming a crucial part of the vibrant cultural legacy.

In the region, healing paths are influenced by the understanding of sickness, derived from identifying and categorizing symptoms. The communities in these lands embrace a collective belief that separates ailments of earthly causes, linked to environmental disharmony, from those of spiritual essence, entwined with societal or divine realms.

Traditional healers harmonize biophysical and symbolic components in their diverse healing techniques. Utilizing incantations, amulets, massages, and herbal remedies tailored to individual contexts, they connect physical ailments to social aspects, preserving cultural and spiritual equilibrium within communities.

Plants

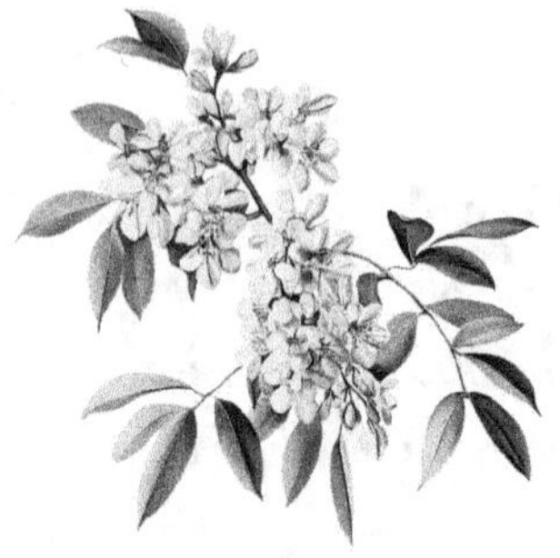

Cassia occidentalis, also known as ***Mbant Maré*** in Wolof, embodies a plant from the Fabaceae family, flourishing across West Africa. Embraced in Senegal to alleviate menstrual cramps, its leaves and roots are crafted into a decoction for their anti-inflammatory and analgesic virtues.

Anastatica hierochuntica, referred to as ***Chajarat Mariam*** in Mauritania, is a desert plant embraced by women for its natural properties in balancing the menstrual cycle and easing discomfort. This plant, representing fertility with its revitalizing and unfolding qualities, plays a significant role in rituals promoting reproductive well-being and purification.

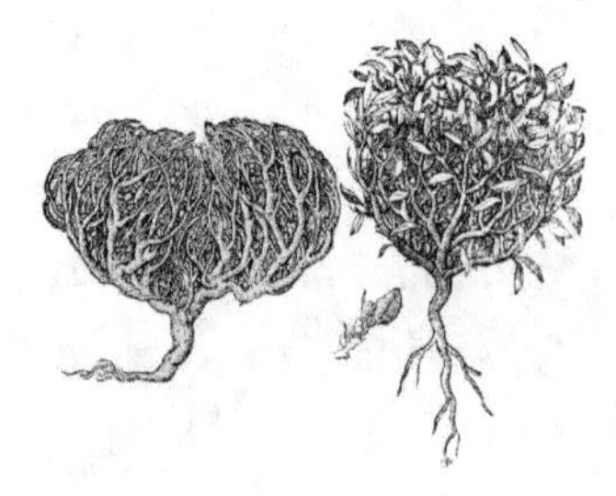

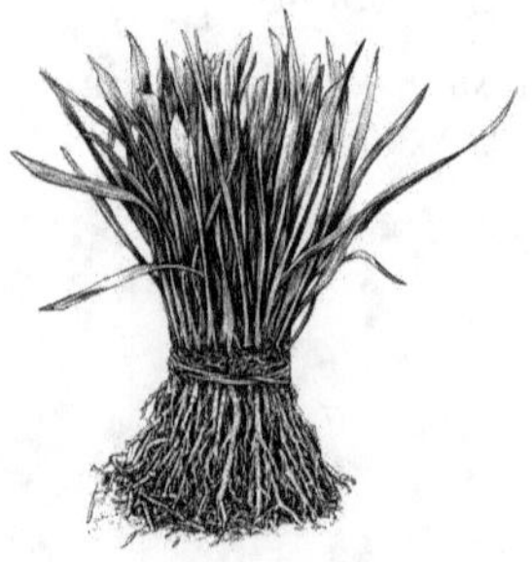

Vetiveria nigritana, known as ***Khamaré*** in Mali, is a plant with roots that Malian women use to ease menstrual discomfort. They create infusions of Khamaré to benefit from its antispasmodic qualities, fostering relaxation and tranquility during this phase of the cycle.

Khamaré Infusion

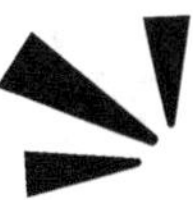

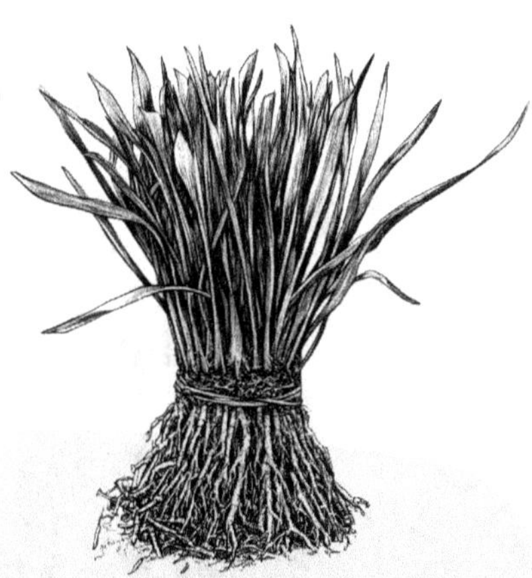

REFRESHING ELIXIR:

- Gather a handful of vetiver stems and immerse them in a container of refreshing water.
- Allow the magic to unfold in the refrigerator for 6 to 8 hours (or overnight).
- Sip and enjoy the infused water all day long for a soothing, revitalizing impact.

WARM ELIXIR:

- Boil water.
- Add a touch of vetiver roots to the simmering water.
- Allow the infusion to steep for 10-15 minutes to intensify its flavor.
- Sip the brewed concoction warm, or allow it to cool before enjoying.

North Africa

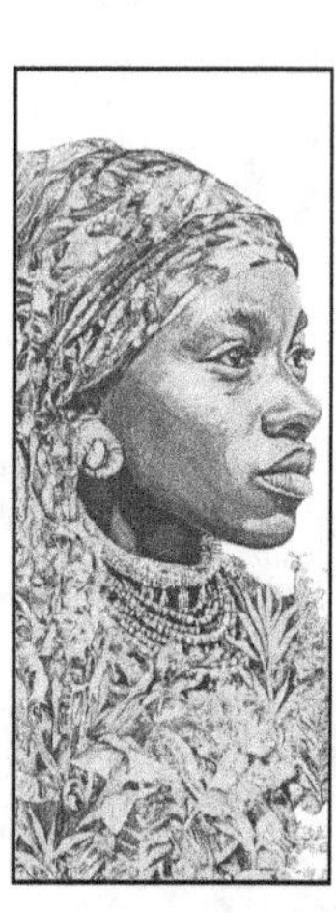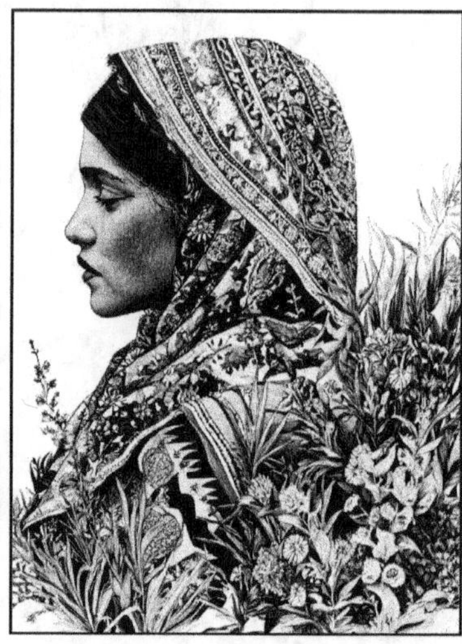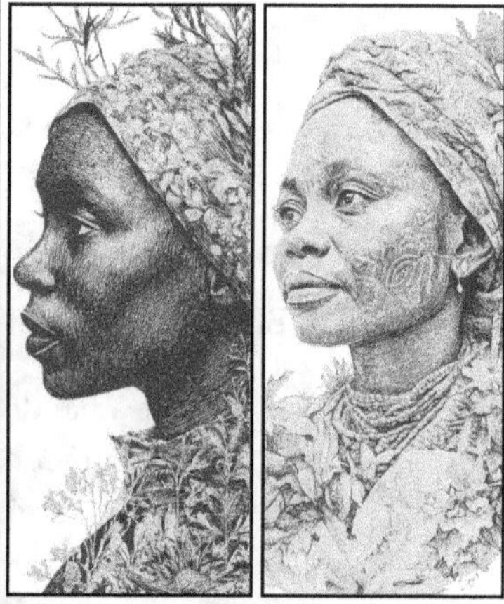

Writing about North Africa and its medicinal traditions is a humble endeavor to grasp the vastness of a millennium-old cultural legacy, a task that may seem insurmountable. This region, stretching from Morocco to Egypt, passing through Algeria and Tunisia, is a fusion of ancient wisdom passed down by women, mirroring the rich cultural tapestry and traditions. Resilience shines brightly amidst modern challenges. Despite urbanization, modernization, and the impact of colonization, these traditional practices hold immense value. In this moment, we celebrate the wisdom of the women we encountered, the protectors of this invaluable legacy.

The Kabyle Spring Festival

*The commemoration of the arrival of spring, known as **Amagger n Tefsut**, embodies an ancient Kabyle custom, firmly entrenched in the Berber heritage of North Africa. Situated in the northern part of Algeria, Kabylia, a region characterized by its mountains, serves as the backdrop for this festivity, signifying the shift from the harsh winter to the rejuvenation of spring. Far from a mere day of observance, this celebration spans several weeks, allowing the Kabyle people to convey their appreciation to the natural world for its abundant gifts. The term Tafsut itself, originating from the Berber root FS(W), conjures images of development and renewal, representing the flourishing of the environment.*

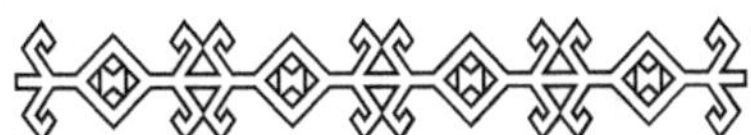

On the brink of the initial day of spring, Kabyle families get ready by gathering thapsia roots (aderyes), a healing plant utilized to create a unique cleansing couscous, *seksu s uderyis*. This dish, which cleanses the body, is crucial for embracing spring in a condition of purity.

The following day, on the day of the celebration, women take on a pivotal role. They adorn themselves in their most exquisite garments, apply makeup, and accompany the children to the fields, bearing pancakes (tiɣrifin) as a gift to the spring. Young girls who have recently had their first menstruation, marking their passage into adulthood, are particularly highlighted. They participate in symbolic rites, such as rolling in the fresh grass, a gesture that seals their communion with nature and which in the past served to designate them as ready for marriage. This rite can, however, vary according to region: in some places, menstruating women are considered to possess disruptive energy and must not touch the earth.

The Kabyle Spring Festival embodies more than just a tribute to nature; it symbolizes the perpetuation and sharing of cultural heritage. *Lalla Tafsut*, the embodiment of spring, epitomizes fertility and renewal. Through timeless songs, rituals, and offerings, the Kabyle community strengthens its identity and unity across generations.

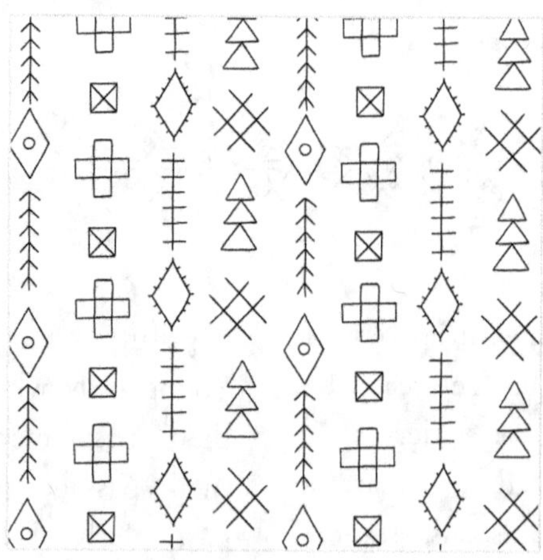

In this celebration, every gesture, every ritual, contributes to a worldview where humanity is in harmony with nature, honoring its cycles and gifts. Therefore, *Amagger n Tefsut* endures as a vibrant tradition, persevering against the challenges to its continuity, and persisting in its crucial role in preserving the intangible cultural legacy of the Kabyles.

Plants

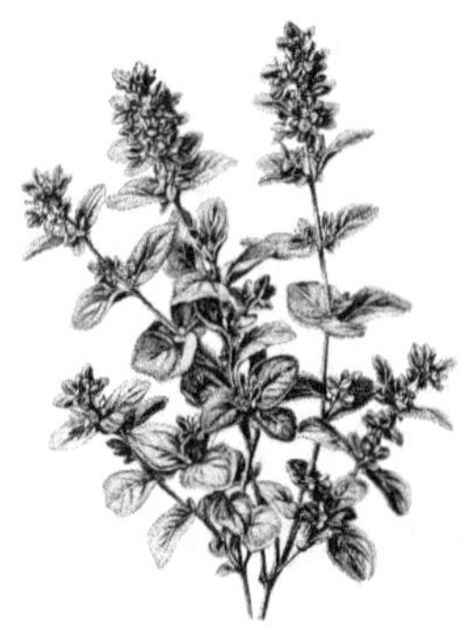

In the northern region of Morocco, ***Origanum vulgare (Origanum vulgare)*** is utilized to alleviate challenging periods. Women create a decoction from the leafy stems of the plant to ease menstrual discomfort.

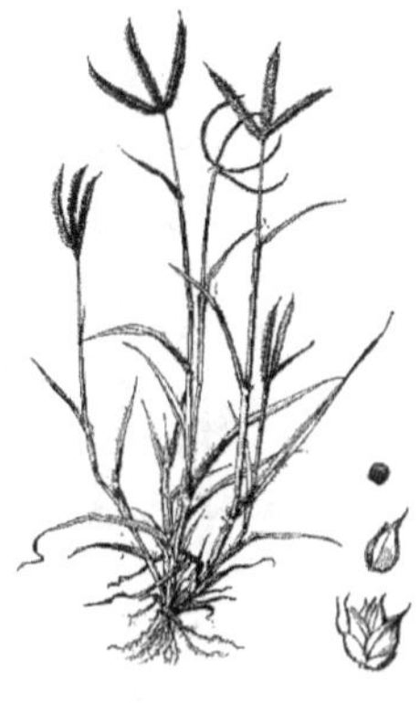

In this very area, ***Dactyloctenium aegyptium or Couch grass***, a wild plant, is conventionally employed to ease discomfort during periods. A concoction made from its rhizome, frequently mixed with asparagus (Asparagus officinalis L.), is utilized to ease these aches. This solution is also applied in addressing female sterility.

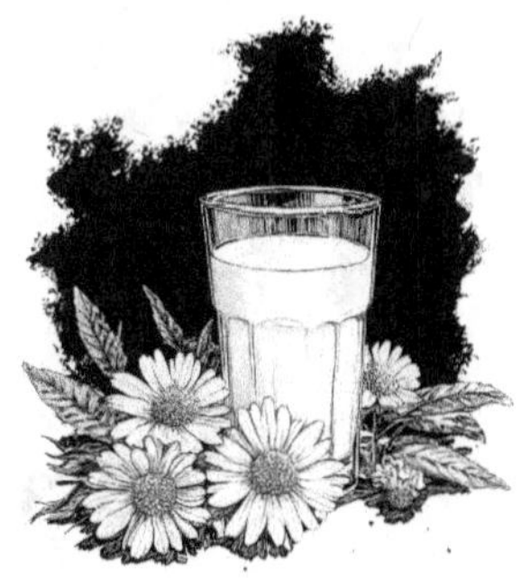

In the areas of Tangier, Chefchaouen, Fifi, and Bab Taza, ***Matricaria chamomilla, German chamomile,*** is a widely utilized plant known for its healing qualities. The blossoms are brewed into a soothing infusion, commonly enjoyed with water or milk, offering relief for discomfort during periods, aiding in digestive issues, and easing migraines. Beyond these purposes, the plant serves as a refreshing mouth rinse.

Argan Oil Massage

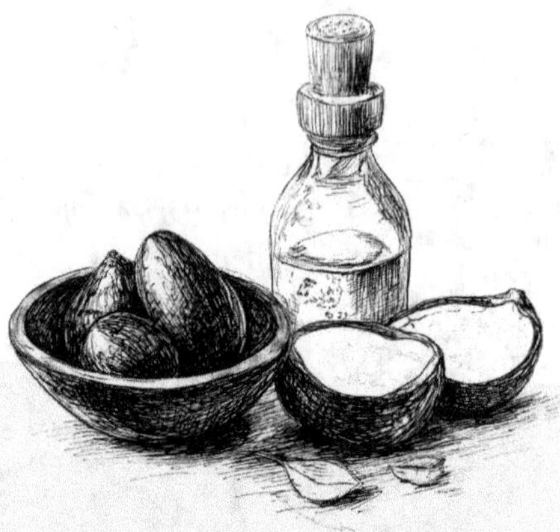

PREPARATION

- Embrace the pure essence of high-quality argan oil, ideally organic. Gently warm a couple of drops of this precious oil between your palms.

APPLICATION

- Pour a few drops of oil into your palm and gently apply it to the lower abdomen. Massage in circular motions around the navel, gradually expanding the circles outwards with light pressure. Keep going for approximately 10 to 15 minutes.

Experience the magic of an argan oil massage, a natural and traditional Moroccan remedy that eases menstrual discomfort while enhancing relaxation and overall wellness.

Infusion of absinthe leaves

Absinthe (*Artemisia absinthium*), locally known as "chiba", holds a significant place in traditional Moroccan medicine, particularly among Berber communities. This hardy plant, often found in the country's mountainous and arid regions, is highly valued for its therapeutic properties and cultural symbolism.

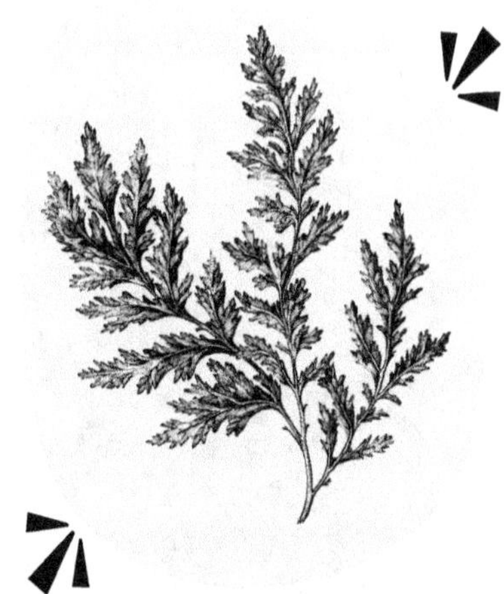

A KNOWLEDGE PASSED DOWN BY BERBER WOMEN

In Berber villages, women have long been the keepers of medicinal knowledge, using local plants to treat various ailments. Absinthe is one of the most commonly used plants for menstrual pain and digestive disorders. Preparing an absinthe infusion is often accompanied by precise gestures and rituals passed down from mother to daughter, illustrating the deep connection between women and nature.

Traditionally, women harvest absinthe at dawn, when its medicinal properties are believed to be at their peak. The leaves are then dried in the shade to preserve their active compounds, before being used as an infusion or decoction depending on the need. This preparation is also shared among neighbors or family members, helping to strengthen community bonds.

HOW TO PREPARE
A TRADITIONAL ABSINTHE INFUSION?

- **Ingredients**:
  - 1 to 2 teaspoons of dried absinthe leaves
  - 250 ml (1 cup) of boiling water
- **Preparation**: Boil the water, add the absinthe leaves, and let them steep, covered, for 5 to 10 minutes. Strain before drinking.
- **Consumption**: Drink one cup, up to three times a day, during menstrual pain. Sweeten with honey to soften the taste.

PRECAUTIONS

- *Absinthe is potent and should not be consumed in excess or for extended periods.*
- *It is contraindicated for pregnant or breastfeeding women and for individuals with neurological or liver disorders.*
- *Always consult a healthcare professional before use, especially if you are taking medications.*

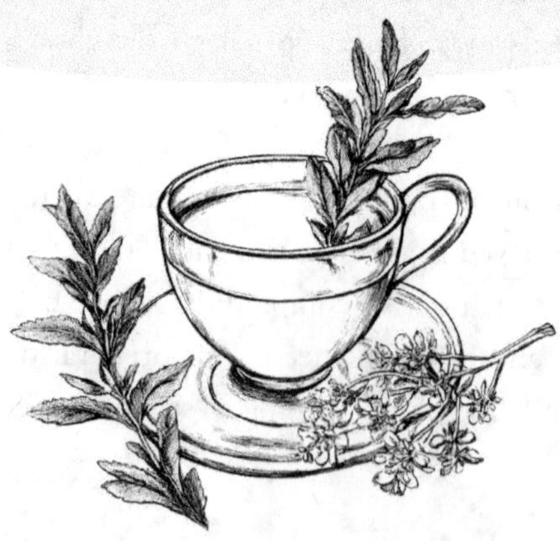

Ancient Egyptian Papyrus

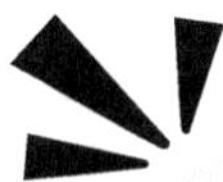

In ancient Egypt, women utilized softened papyrus, a grass-like aquatic plant, to absorb their menstrual flow. These primitive tampons symbolize one of the earliest known historical accounts of menstrual management.

Papyrus stems were cut, softened, and then rolled or folded to create a type of pad. This plant material, though basic, proved quite efficient in its era, owing to its absorbent qualities.

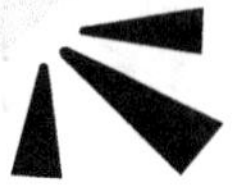

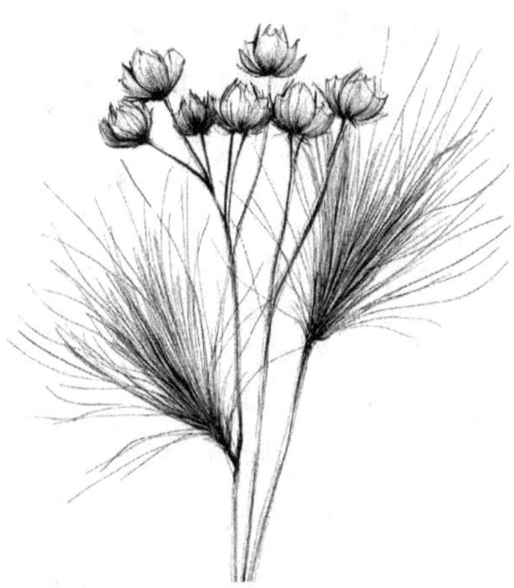

Great Lakes Region

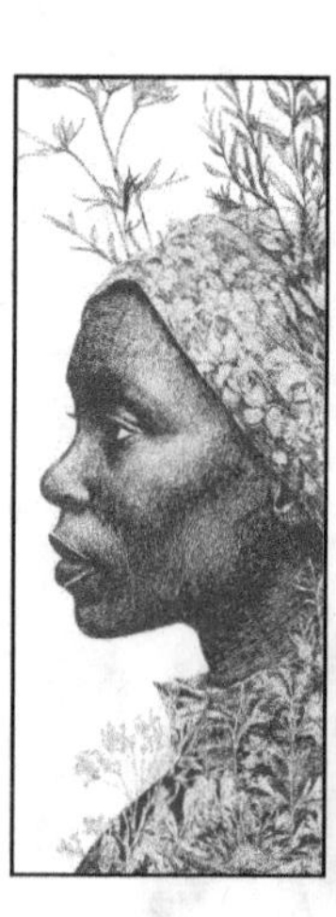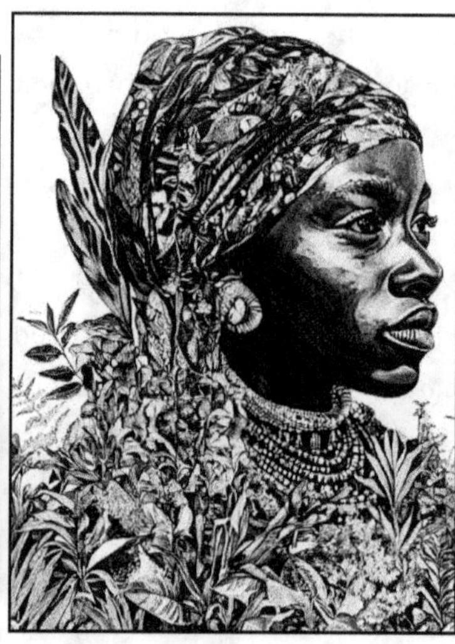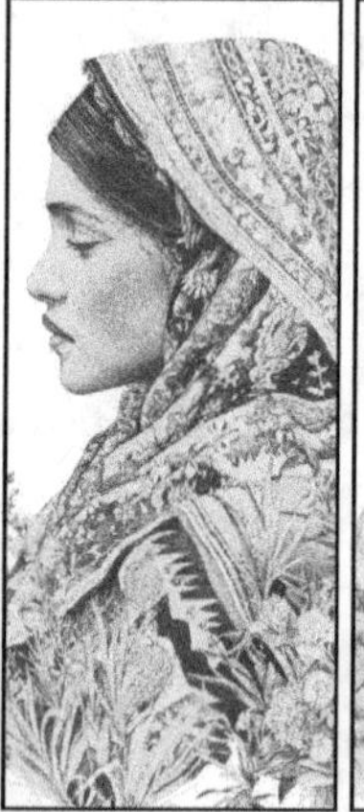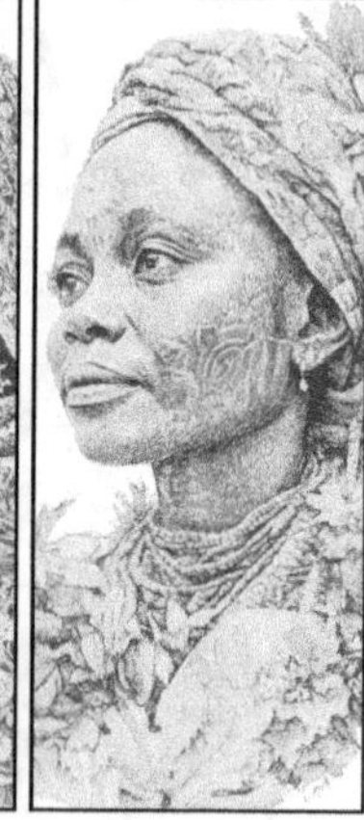

The Great Lakes Region of Africa, situated predominantly around Lakes Victoria, Tanganyika, and Albert, embodies extraordinary natural and cultural richness. It embraces remarkable ethnic diversity, with communities that have coexisted for centuries.

Evolved with extraordinary natural and cultural riches, the Great Lakes Region is a place of remarkable ethnic diversity, where communities have harmoniously co-evolved with the natural surroundings for generations.

Traditions

The communities of the Great Lakes Region have cultivated intricate ancestral wisdom concerning the utilization of healing plants, farming, and the preservation of woodland ecosystems, empowering them to thrive in diverse landscapes, from mountains to lush plains.

Nevertheless, the area is currently encountering numerous challenges, such as deforestation, excessive use of natural resources, and climate change, all of which are endangering this delicate equilibrium. Moreover, ethnic tensions and violent conflicts, frequently intensified by the competition for natural resources control, have characterized the region's recent past, resulting in the displacement of populations and enduring social unrest.

In this segment, our attention shifts to Kenya, a land of extraordinary diversity, both culturally and botanically. With more than forty unique ethnic communities such as the Kikuyu, Luhya, Luo, and Maasai, each contributing their distinct traditions and languages, the nation presents a captivating cultural tapestry. This cultural abundance resonates in the nation's botanical variety, encompassing over seven thousand native plant species thriving in diverse ecosystems, ranging from rainforests to savannahs.

The ancestral wisdom regarding the healing properties of these plants, transmitted through ages, embodies a valuable legacy.

Discover the Kalenjin

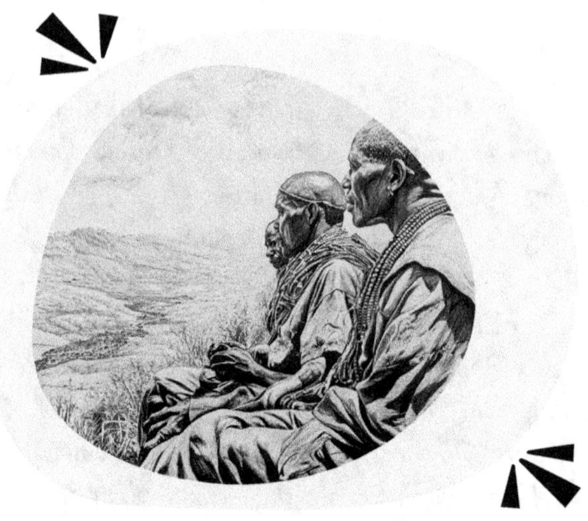

The Kalenjin, a vibrant East African community rooted in the former Rift Valley Province of Kenya, possess a profound heritage of ancestral healing. Within their culture, the revered healers, known as "doctors," exhibit extraordinary mystical abilities to identify and address the roots of adversity or ailment. Conversely, female herbalists and midwives draw upon their expertise in practical wisdom. The Kalenjin healing practices embrace both the mystical and practical dimensions. Ailments are frequently linked to restless spirits, necessitating cleansing rituals prior to therapy. Healing concoctions are meticulously crafted from an array of barks, roots, and foliage.

This comprehensive method of healing embodies the profound wisdom of ancestral Kalenjin medicine, transmitted across generations.

Syzygium Guineense Infusion

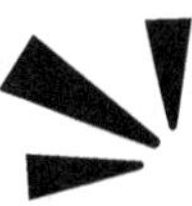

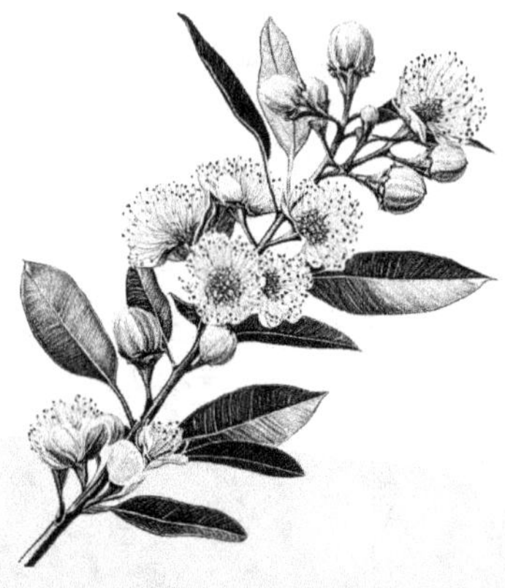

PREPARATION

- Gather 100g of vibrant bark from the stem of Syzygium guinneense.
- Immerse the bark in 1 liter of chilly water for the night.
- The following day, strain the brew.

DOSAGE

- Consume 250 ml of this elixir thrice daily until signs of improvement manifest.

PRECAUTIONS

Syzygium guineense, a tree from the Myrtaceae family, hails from Africa. The Nandi people, a part of the Kalenjin group, have long revered its bark for its healing qualities. This ancient remedy has been carefully recorded through ethnobotanical studies. It is advisable to seek guidance from a healthcare provider prior to usage.

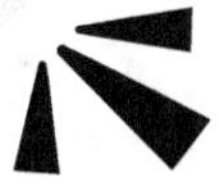

Indian Ocean Islands

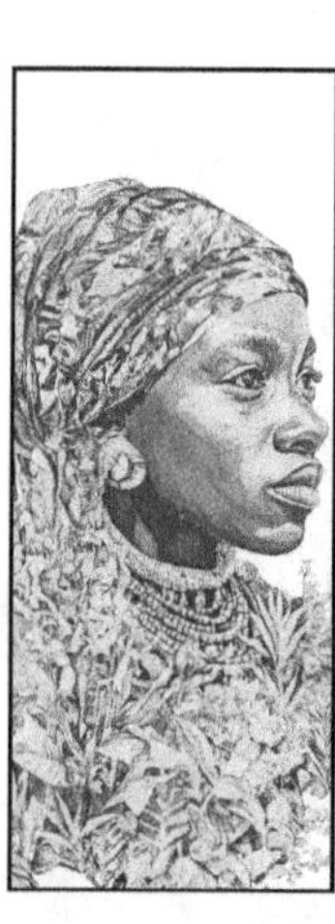
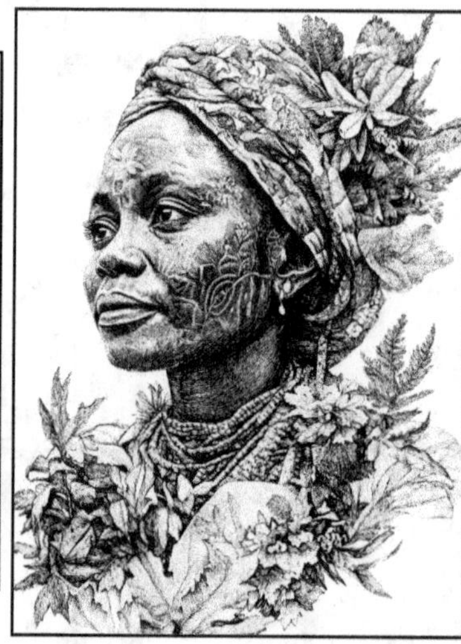
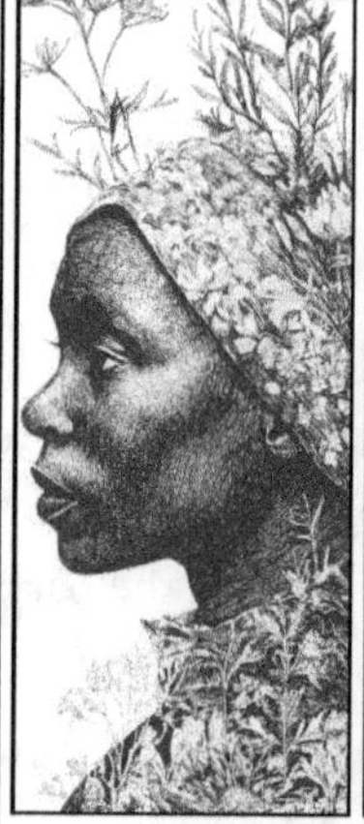
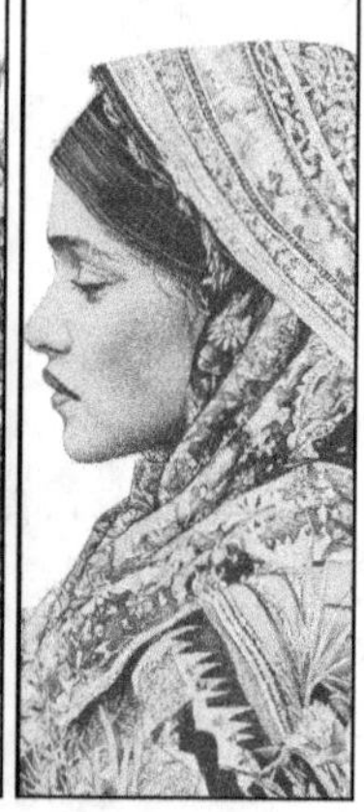

The islands of the Indian Ocean hold a treasure trove of traditional wisdom, especially nurtured by women. This wisdom, a product of centuries of history and cultural fusion, surpasses the varied origins of the populations - Malagasy, Indian, African, Asian, and European - who have inhabited these islands.

Over time, connections among these diverse communities have sparked a collective legacy of wisdom, transcending social or ethnic boundaries. This ancestral wisdom is not stagnant but continuously grows, mirroring the vibrancy of island societies.

Plants

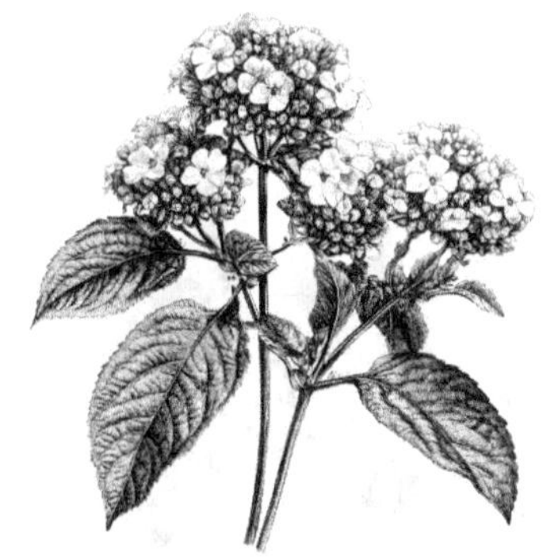

In Mayotte, the exotic plant **Lantana camara**, known locally as **Sari fatsiki madani** in Kibushi, is utilized for preparing different remedies by crushing and boiling it. To regulate the menstrual cycle in the event of frequent periods, a mixture of the roots and fruits of Lantana camara, along with the fruit of Alangium salviifolium (mgiligi in Shimaoré), is administered.

Tetikampu, a traditional remedy from the Comoros region, is a magical solution for easing discomfort during periods. It involves a special decoction made from the bark of the **Heritiera littoralis** tree, also known as murumuni or mukomafii locally. The bark is carefully collected from the tree's eastern side at the break of dawn. This enchanting decoction is to be savored three times daily. Yet, its enchanting powers call for careful consideration, especially among young maidens, as it may influence their future fertility.

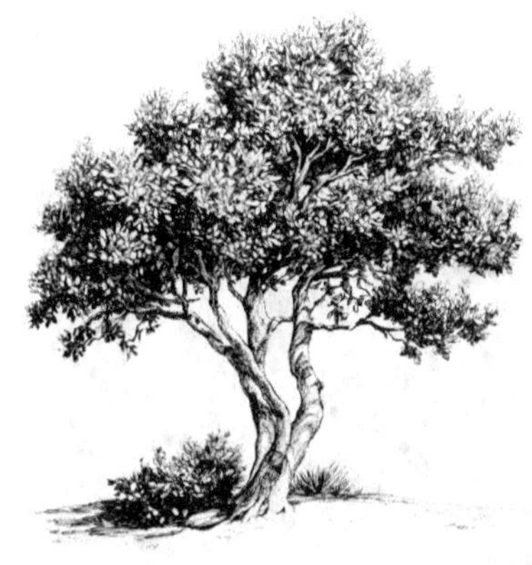

Zerbages Péi from Reunion Island

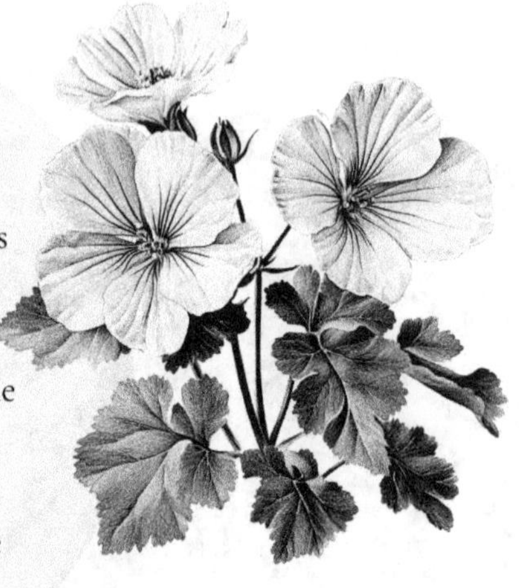

Péi plants embody the essence of the island of Reunion, being either endemic or traditionally utilized. This term in Creole typically denotes indigenous plants with cultural, medicinal, or culinary significance. The diverse flora of Reunion, flourishing with numerous endemic species, is a result of the island's seclusion and the wide range of microclimates it hosts.

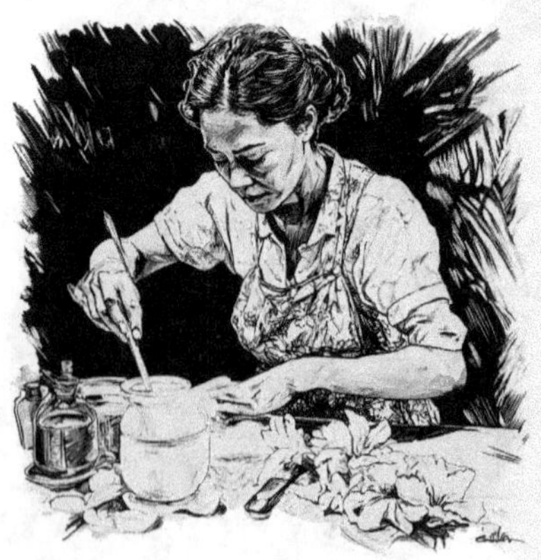

Thanks to its potent antispasmodic properties, *Bourbon geranium* essential oil brings relief to colitis, stomach aches, intestinal spasms, uterine contractions, and menstrual pain. To experience its benefits, blend geranium essential oil with a vegetable oil, a hydrosol, a natural extract, or infuse it into food, a bath, or an essential oil diffuser.

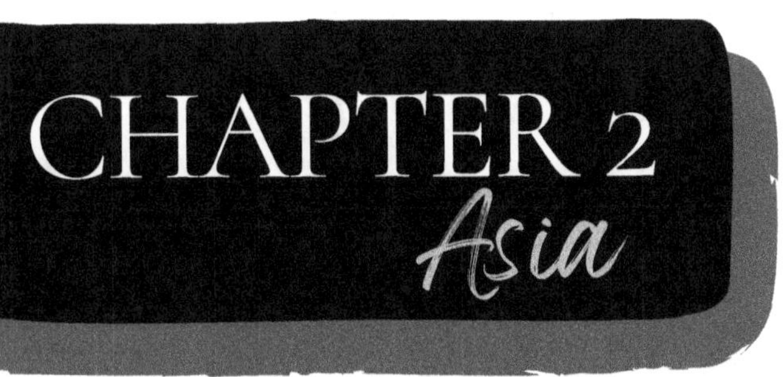

INDIA

INDONESIA

CHINA

JAPAN

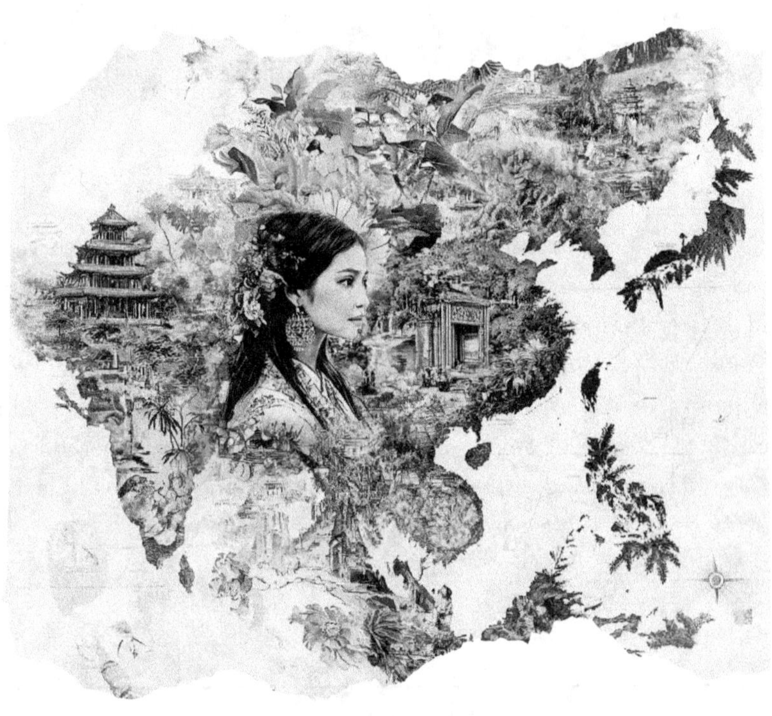

India

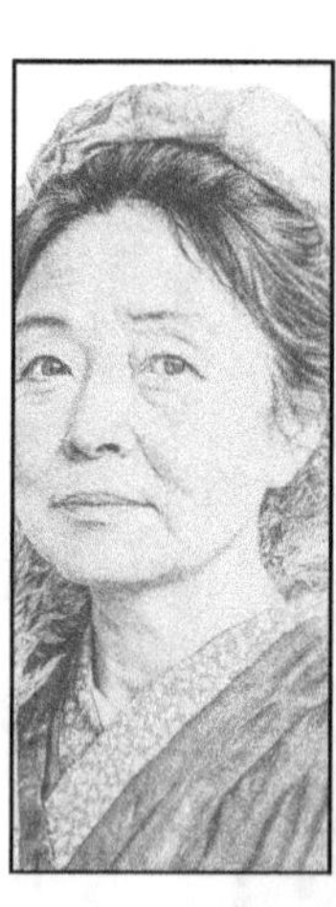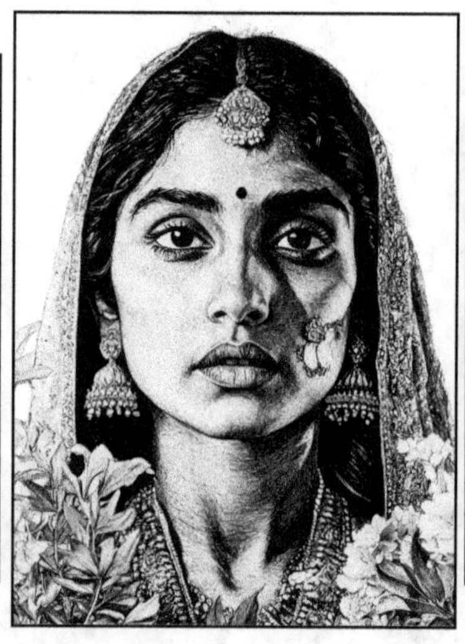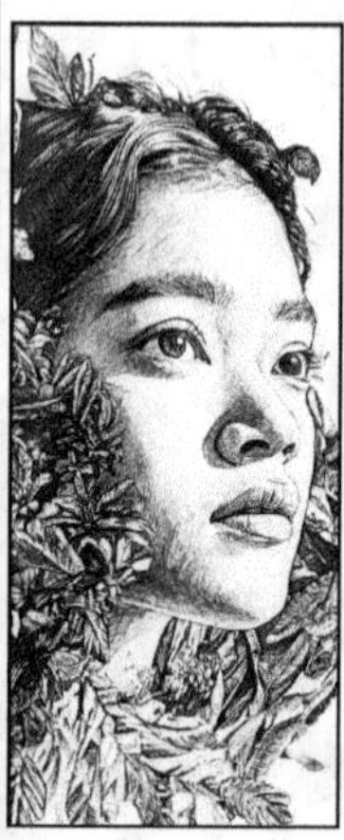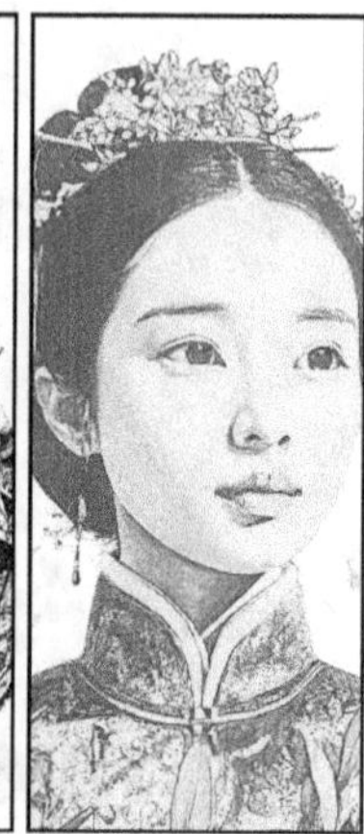

In India, menstruation is enveloped by diverse traditions and beliefs that differ based on regions and communities. It is commonly viewed as a period of cleansing, yet also of stigma and seclusion, prompting women to take a break to safeguard their essential energy, Ojas, and Ayurveda. The ancient Ayurvedic medicine, with over five thousand years of wisdom, holds a pivotal role in comprehending and addressing menstrual pain, providing holistic methods to harmonize the cycle and alleviate women's symptoms.

The Sari Ceremony

In India, especially within the Hindu communities of South India, the Ritu Kala Samskaram ceremony, also known as the Sari ceremony or *Langa Voni*, is a ritual that signifies the transition from childhood to adulthood for girls.

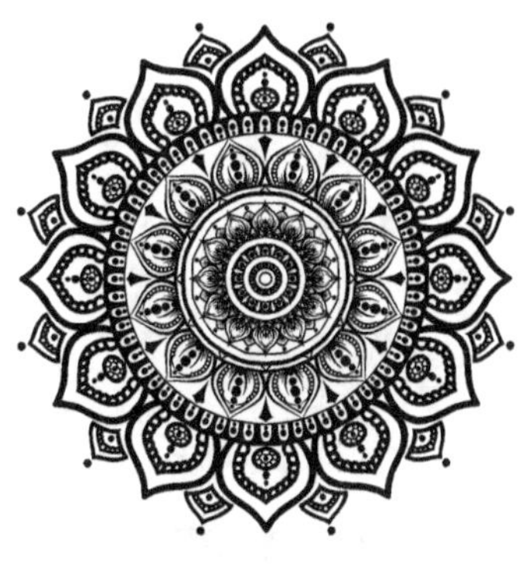

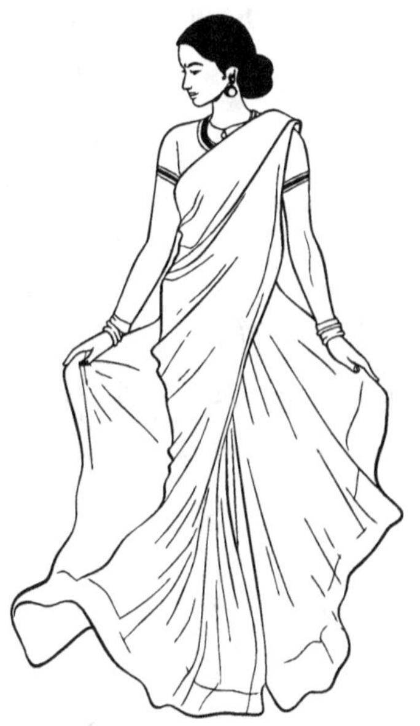

Celebrate the significant moment when a girl experiences her first period, signifying her journey into womanhood. Embrace the tradition where she receives her inaugural half-sari or Langa Voni, a symbolic attire. This garment will adorn her until the day of her wedding, where she will gracefully transition to a one-piece sari, marking another pivotal moment in her life's journey.

Ayurvedic Medicine

Ayurveda perceives menstruation as a vital component of the natural life cycle, shaped by the doshas (Vata, Pitta, Kapha), which are essential energies in the human body.

Every dosha has the power to impact menstrual cycles uniquely, and any disharmony can result in the discomfort known as Kashta Artava.

- Excess of **Vata**, the energy of movement, can lead to spasmodic pain and cramps. It is commonly addressed through calming methods like gentle oil massages, warmth on the lower abdomen, and consuming a nurturing diet filled with warm, sweet, and mildly spicy foods.

- Embrace the essence of **Pitta**, linked with warmth and change. When this energy is in harmony, it radiates balance and vitality. However, when imbalance arises, it may surface as heat, discomfort, and heightened sensitivity. To nurture Pitta, consider the wisdom of Ayurveda. Explore the realm of cooling nourishment, savor herbal infusions such as fennel and coriander, and embrace calming rituals like meditation.

- Look for balance within **Kapha** to avoid stagnation and heaviness, experiencing lightness and vitality. Incorporate remedies like nourishing foods, invigorating spices like ginger, and soothing movements to promote circulation.

Traditional Healing Methods

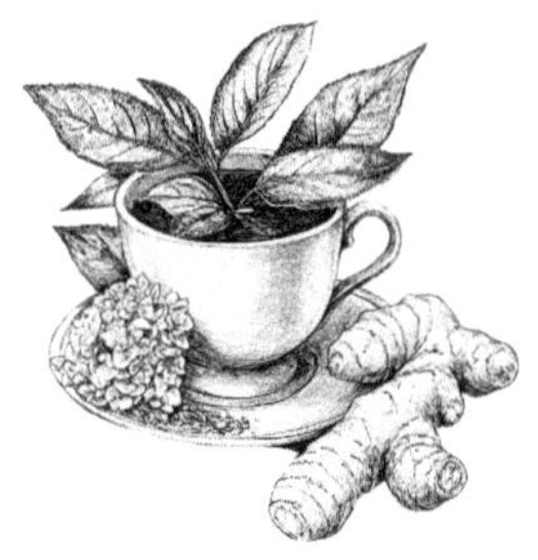

ELIXIRS AND BREWS

Herbs such as **Ashwagandha, Shatavari,** ginger, and turmeric are commonly utilized to harmonize the menstrual cycle and alleviate discomfort.

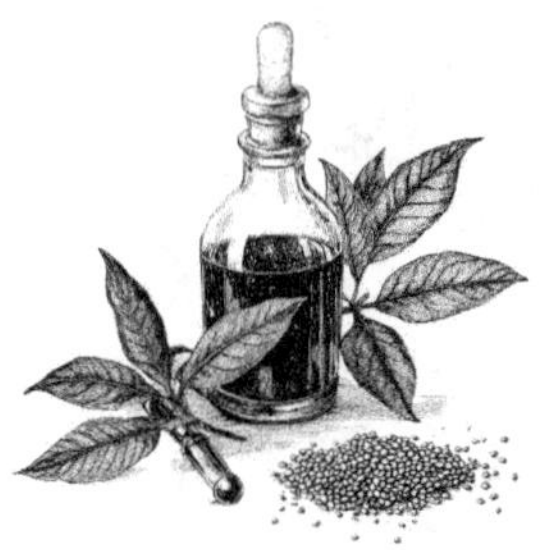

SOOTHING OIL MASSAGES

Soothing **Sesame oils**, occasionally blended with special herbs, are used in massages to alleviate spasms and unwind muscles.

DIET

Focus on nourishing foods that harmonize the doshas, paying special attention to warmth, lightness, and effortless digestion throughout menstruation.

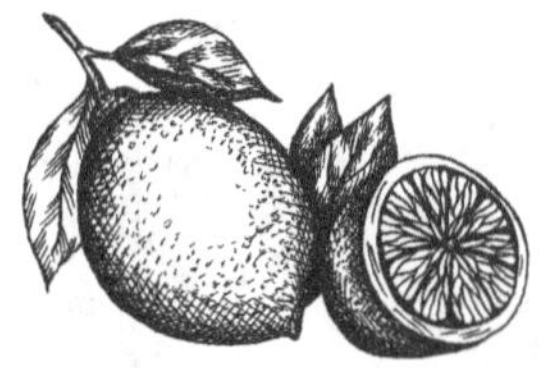

EMOTIONAL WELLNESS

Ayurveda emphasizes nurturing the mind and emotions during menstruation. Engaging in gentle yoga, meditation, and purification rituals is advised to promote mental equilibrium and alleviate stress, which may intensify menstrual discomfort.

Warm Sesame Oil Massage

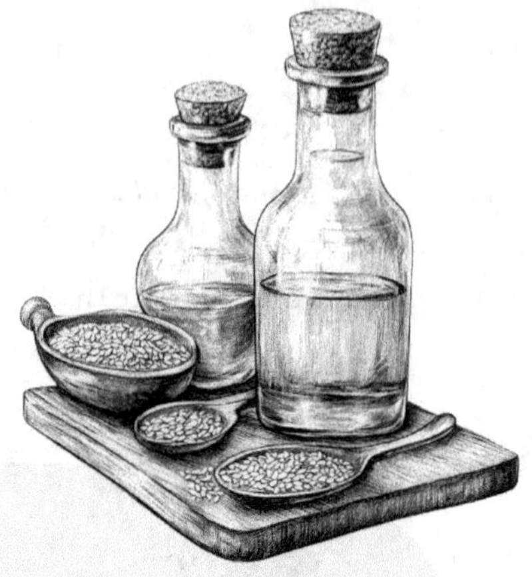

PREPARATION OF WARM OIL
- Gently heat 2 to 3 tablespoons of sesame oil in a bowl (preferably using a double boiler to avoid excessive heat). The oil should be warm, never hot.

APPLICATION
- Gently massage the lower abdomen with the warm oil, using circular motions in a clockwise direction. This movement follows the natural flow of the organs and promotes relaxation.
- Continue the massage for 10 to 15 minutes to allow the oil to penetrate deeply.

ENHANCED EFFECT WITH WARM COMPRESSES
- After the massage, place a warm towel or a hot water bottle on the lower abdomen to intensify the benefits of the oil.

Indonesia

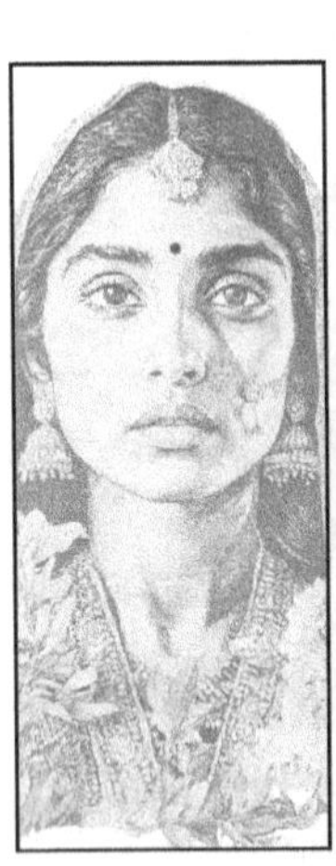
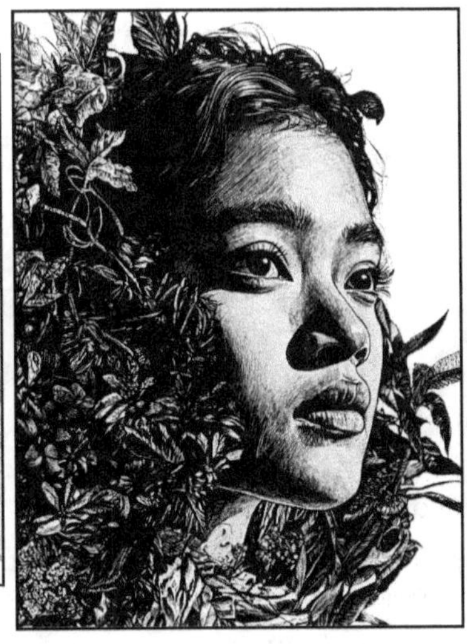
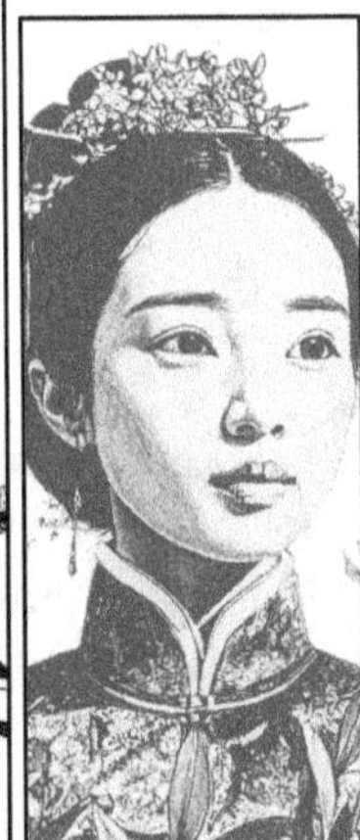
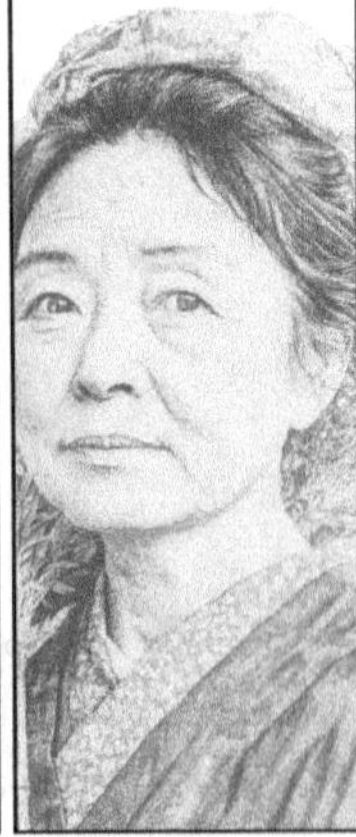

Indonesia, a vast archipelago comprising thousands of islands, stands as a meeting point of cultures, ethnicities, and ancient customs. Every region, from Sumatra to Bali through Java, holds its own inherited wisdom, transmitted through the ages. Traditions lie at the core of conserving natural remedies and healing practices, passed down from the cultural diversity of their numerous ethnic groups. This wisdom, ingrained in daily life, mirrors the balance between humanity, nature, and the spiritual realm, providing a comprehensive outlook on wellness.

Plants

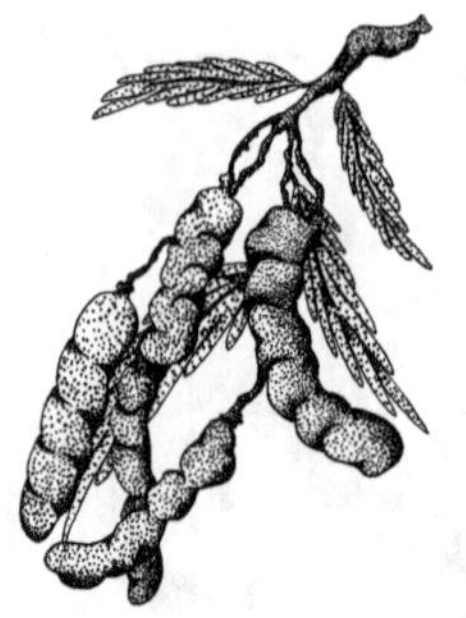

Tamarind, Tamarindus indica, or *Asem* in Bahasa Indonesia, serves not only in culinary delights but also as a healing elixir. A concoction made from asem pulp blended with warm water is believed to soothe the soul and alleviate stomach discomfort linked to menstruation.

Turmeric, known as *Kunyit* (Curcuma longa), serves as a healing solution for alleviating menstrual cramps. Cultivated in lush, fertile lands, this tropical plant is transformed into a paste named boreh kunyit. By grinding the turmeric roots and blending them with water or oil, this paste, when applied to the lower abdomen, diminishes inflammation and eases menstrual cramps, all thanks to the curcumin within.

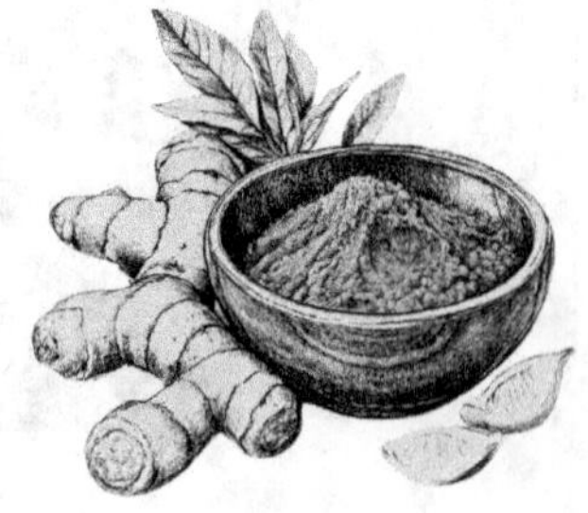

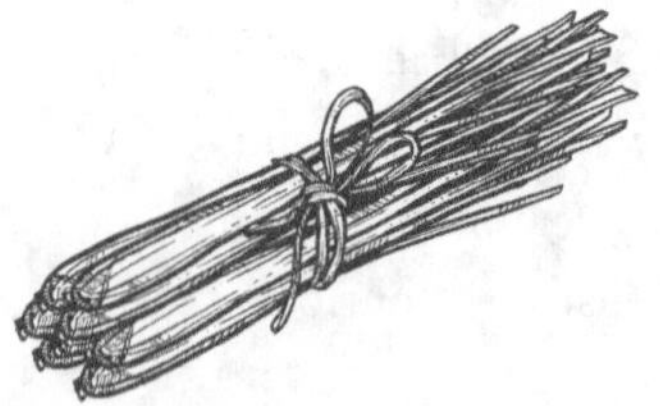

Lemongrass, also known as *Serai*, is a tropical herb with muscle relaxant properties. It is commonly used in cooking. A soothing sera tea made by boiling its stems is a traditional remedy for relieving menstrual pain.

Betel Leaf Compresses

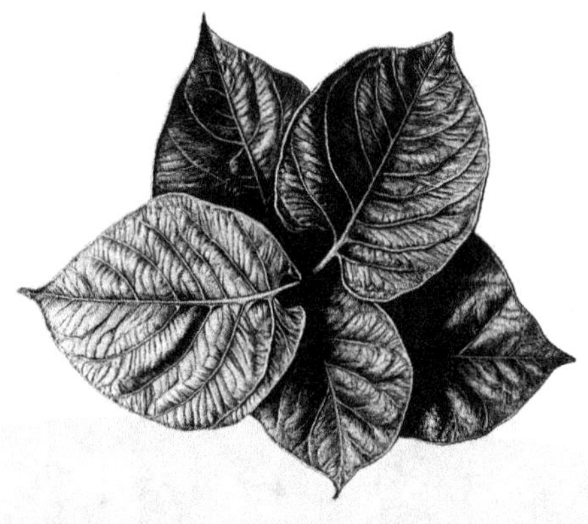

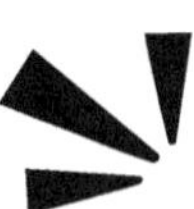

*Regarded as sacred and frequently utilized in different purification ceremonies, betel leaves, known as **Daun sirih** in the native tongue, are a customary treatment valued for their pain-relieving qualities.*

INDICATIONS

- Delicately warm 2 to 3 betel leaves over a flame or immerse them in hot water for a few seconds.

- Apply the warm leaves directly to the lower belly.

- Wrap with a cloth to preserve warmth.

- Let it stay for 15 to 20 minutes, reapplying if needed.

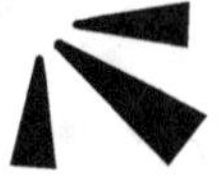

China

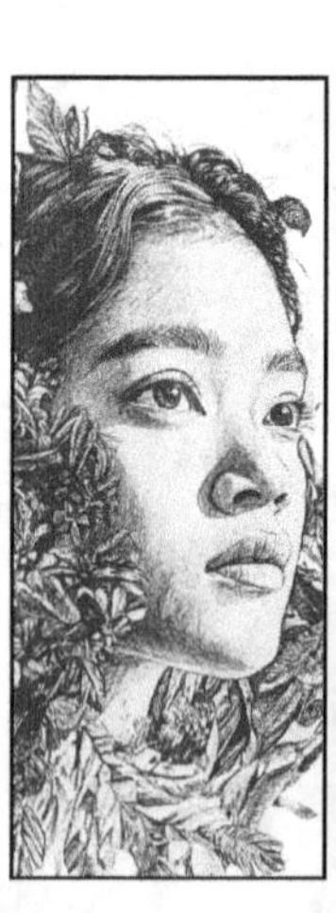

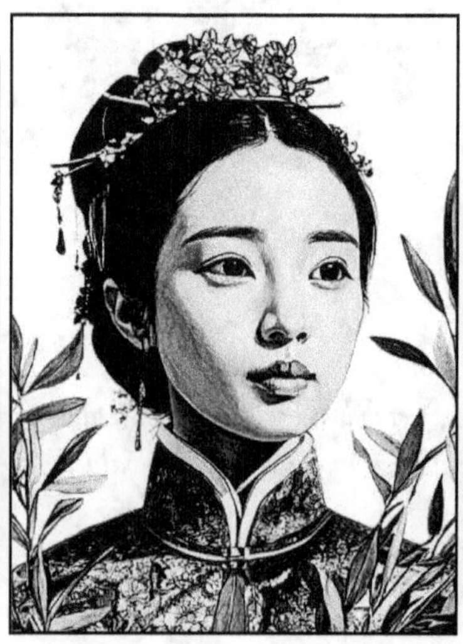

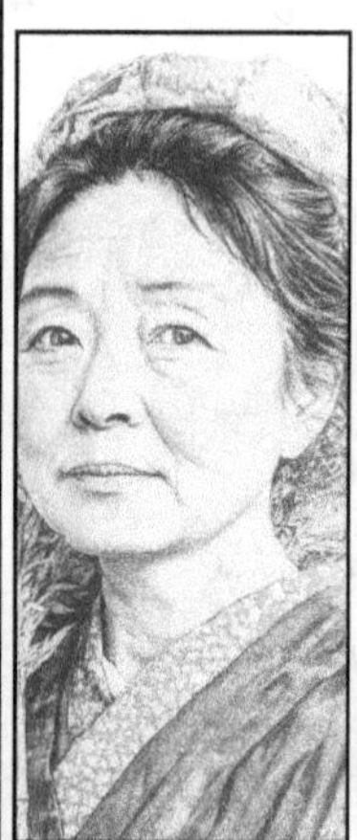

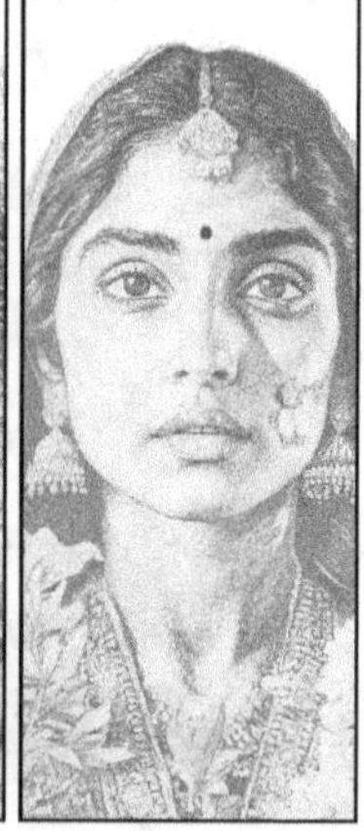

In China, menstruation is viewed as a natural phenomenon, yet frequently shrouded in taboos and secrecy, particularly in traditional settings. This phase is considered a period when the body is more delicate, necessitating specific attention to preserve the Qi (vital energy), revitalize energy and maintain balance. The transition into womanhood is celebrated with intimate family traditions and guidance. These traditions encompass suggestions on nutrition, relaxation, and cleanliness, to uphold equilibrium of energy and avert potential discomfort or issues.

Chinese Medicine

Traditional Chinese medicine has a significant impact on addressing menstrual symptoms in China, with a history of practice spanning thousands of years. In this approach, menstruation is viewed as more than just a physical process; it is seen as a harmonious interplay of Qi, blood, and internal organs, notably the kidneys, liver, and spleen. These vital organs are pivotal in maintaining the balance of the menstrual cycle and promoting holistic reproductive well-being.

In the realm of traditional Chinese medicine, the menstrual cycle embodies the harmonious interplay of Qi and blood. The liver plays a crucial role in the flow of Qi and blood throughout the body. Any disruption in its function can result in stagnation, giving rise to menstrual discomfort, irregularities, or cramping. Likewise, the kidneys are linked to vitality and fertility, and any deficiency may lead to scanty or absent menstruation. The spleen contributes to blood formation, and its impairment can trigger fatigue and excessive bleeding. When these vital organs are in disharmony, it may lead to various menstrual issues, including pain, irregular cycles, excessive bleeding, and even more serious problems like infertility. For instance, stagnant Liver Qi can lead to severe menstrual pain, headaches, and mood swings. An imbalance in the Spleen can cause a feeling of heaviness and fatigue during menstruation.

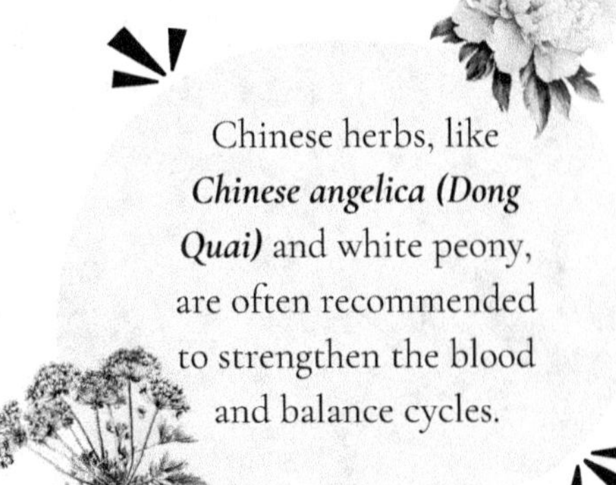

Chinese herbs, like **Chinese angelica (Dong Quai)** and white peony, are often recommended to strengthen the blood and balance cycles.

Acupuncture

Acupuncture seeks to align energies to alleviate symptoms and renew the body's innate harmony.

Harmonization of the Menstrual Cycle

Irregular menstruation can be addressed by activating specific points that harmonize hormones and enhance the functions of the kidney and liver. One such point is the Zigong point (EX-CA1), situated in the lower abdomen, which aids in boosting blood flow to the uterus and fostering consistent menstrual cycles.

Easing Menstrual Discomfort

Acupuncture works wonders in addressing menstrual cramps by targeting specific points that enhance blood circulation and release tense muscles. One key point, the Sanyinjiao point (SP6), situated on the leg, is commonly activated to alleviate menstrual cramps and enhance blood flow in the pelvic region.

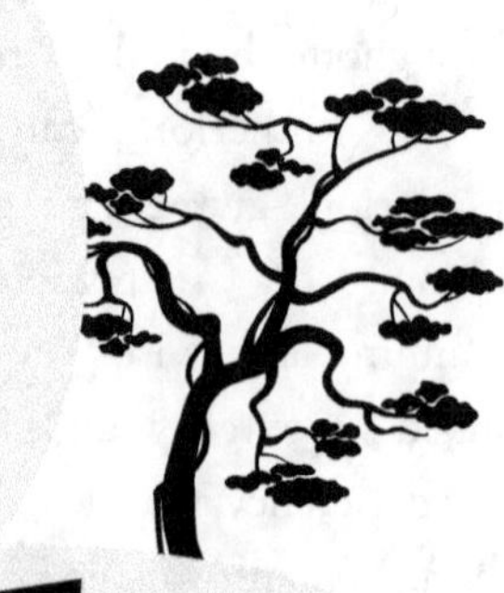

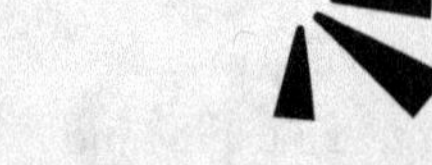

Transformation of Premenstrual Syndrome

By addressing aspects concerning emotional regulation and digestion, acupuncture aids in decreasing inflammation, harmonizing emotions, and removing excess fluids from the body.

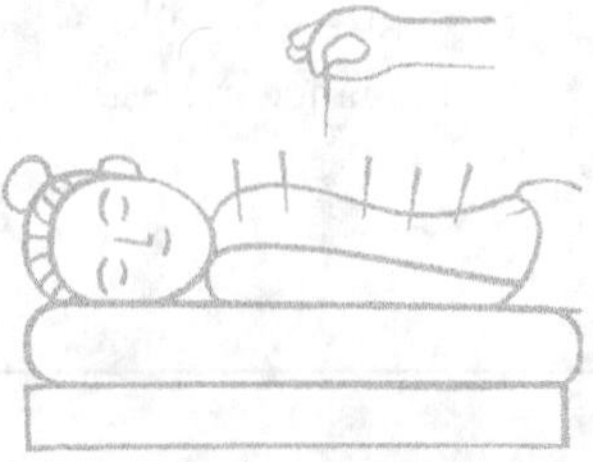

Japan

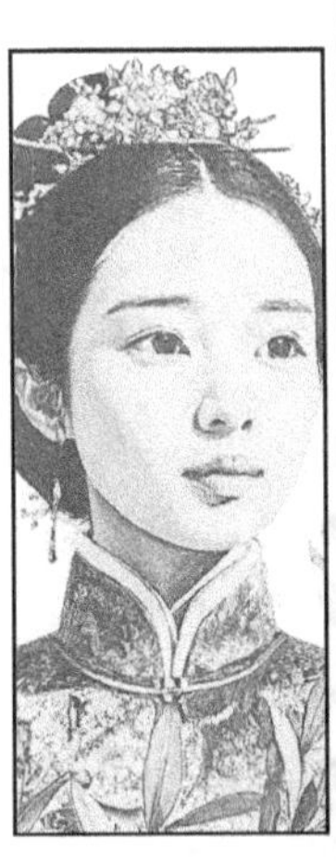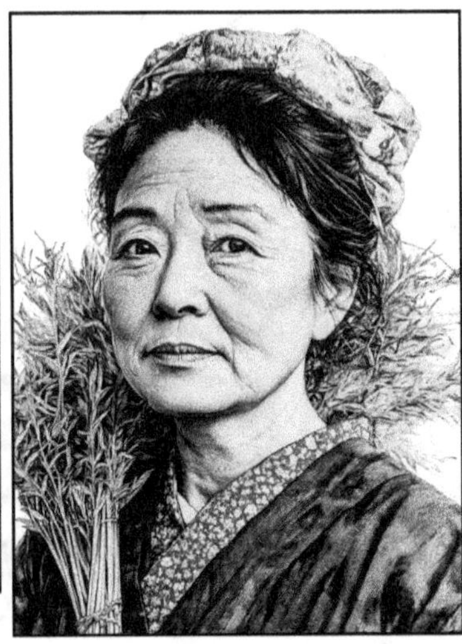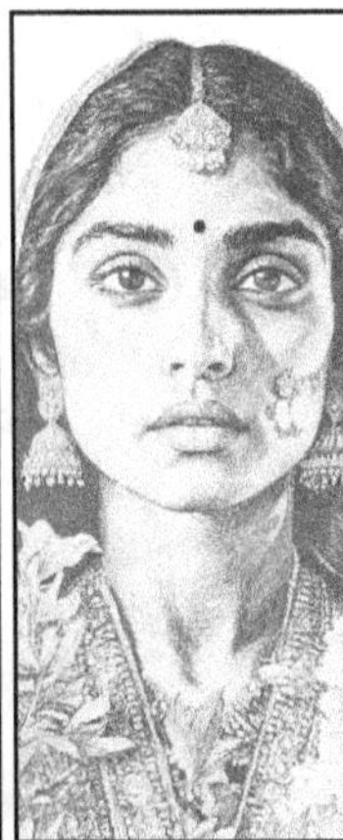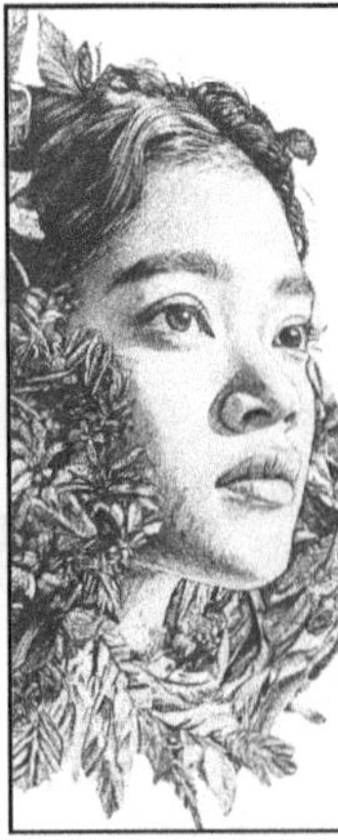

In Japan, menstruation has long been enveloped in taboos, viewed as both a time of purification and temporary impurity, impacting women's involvement in religious and social activities. Nevertheless, these mindsets have shifted, and now menstruation is progressively accepted. The open discussion of menstruation is on the rise, especially through educational initiatives and awareness efforts. Girls are gaining knowledge about the topic starting from primary school. While the subject may have been approached with caution before, it is becoming less of a taboo.

Sekihan Preparation

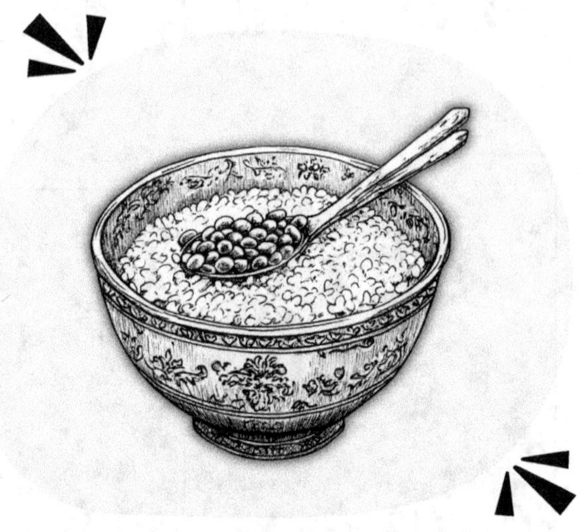

Sekihan, *a traditional Japanese dish made of sticky rice and azuki beans, is frequently cooked to commemorate significant life milestones.*

This vibrant dish is symbolically associated with abundance and joy. In Japan, while conversations about menstruation may be discreet, certain families quietly commemorate a young girl's first period by crafting sekihan.

This act, though not directly mentioned, is perceived as an acknowledgment of the journey into maturity. Sekihan is also presented during various joyous events like birthdays, weddings, and festivities of well-being and success, further solidifying its significance as a representation of joy and abundance in Japanese traditions.

The Art of Shiatsu

Discover the essence of Shiatsu, a profound Japanese healing art that originated in the early 20th century, yet its origins delve even deeper. Rooted in ancient Japanese massage practices like Anma and enriched by the wisdom of traditional Chinese medicine, Shiatsu embodies the power of touch. The very name, Shiatsu, signifies the significance of finger pressure, the cornerstone of this transformative therapy.

Shiatsu draws significant inspiration from traditional Chinese medicine, specifically embracing the notions of meridians (energy channels) and Qi (vital energy). In contrast to acupuncture's use of needles, shiatsu employs manual pressure using fingers, hands, and occasionally elbows and knees. By integrating various physical manipulation methods, shiatsu focuses on a more hands-on approach aimed at enhancing immediate physical wellness.

Shiatsu operates by administering rhythmic pressure to particular points on the body. This pressure aids in invigorating the flow of Qi through the meridians, easing muscles, enhancing blood circulation, and fostering harmony in the body. Apart from addressing particular conditions like muscle pain, headaches, or digestive disorders, shiatsu is also employed to diminish stress, enhance general well-being, and bolster the body's internal functions.

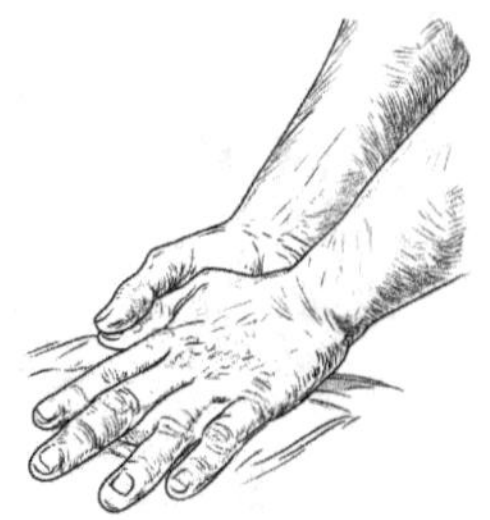

Shiso Tea

In Japan, perilla (*Perilla frutescens*), known as shiso, holds an essential place in traditional Kampo medicine, derived from ancient Chinese medicine. Renowned for its anti-inflammatory and antispasmodic properties, this plant is a cornerstone of natural feminine care. Its use in infusions, particularly popular, helps women soothe menstrual cramps while boosting their immunity.

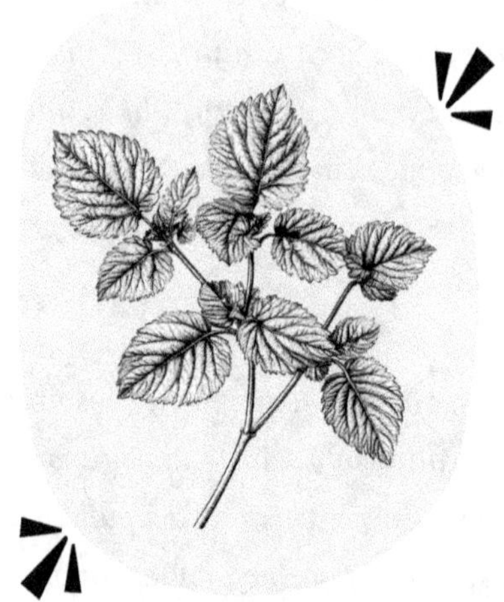

A PLANT AT THE HEART OF JAPANESE TRADITIONS

In Japanese culture, shiso is much more than a remedy. It also symbolizes vitality and longevity. Japanese women have passed down the art of using it for menstrual health from generation to generation. Shiso is often grown in family gardens, a testament to its importance in daily care.

In Kampo medicine, perilla is also prescribed to treat other feminine concerns, such as irregular cycles and menopause symptoms. Its widespread use highlights its key role in women's well-being.

Although shiso is generally safe, it is recommended to consult a healthcare professional in cases of pregnancy or specific allergies.

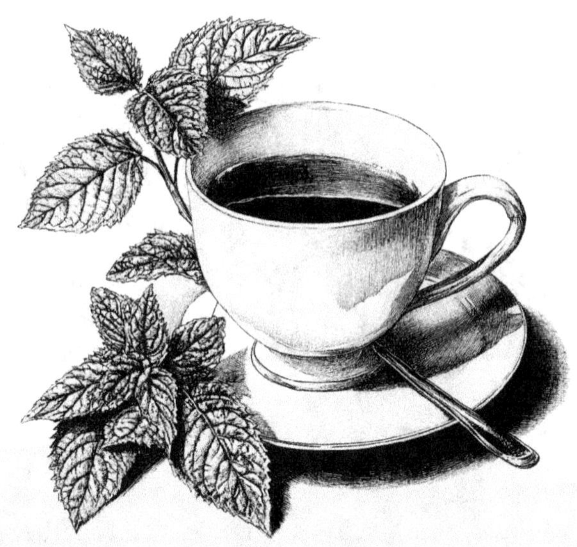

INGREDIENTS
- 1 to 2 teaspoons of dried shiso leaves (red or green)
- 250 ml of hot water (not boiling, around 80°C)

PREPARATION
- Place the leaves in a cup or teapot.
- Pour the hot water over the leaves and let steep for 5 to 7 minutes.
- Strain before drinking.

CONSUMPTION
- Drink 1 to 2 cups per day during menstruation.
- The tea can be lightly sweetened with honey or flavored with ginger to enhance its anti-inflammatory effects.

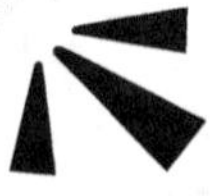

CHAPTER 3
America

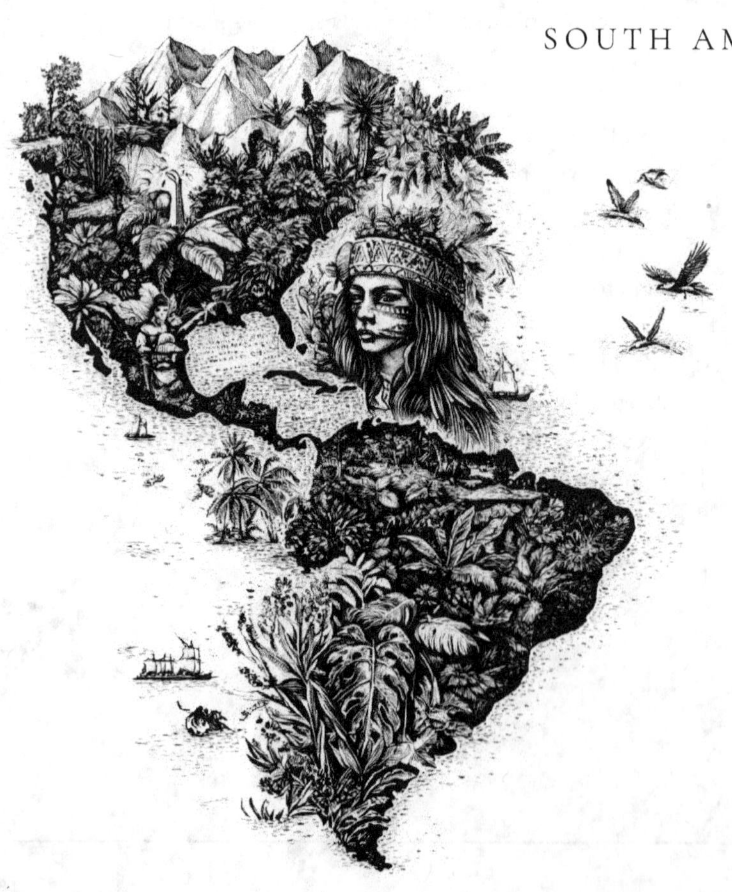

North America

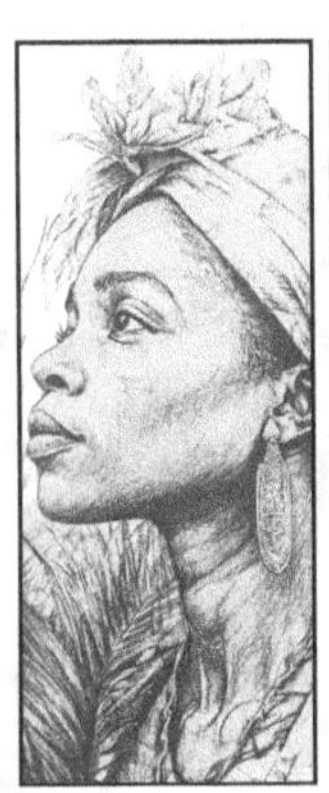 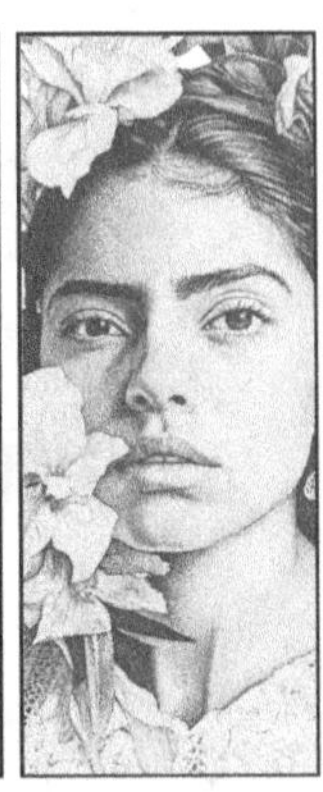 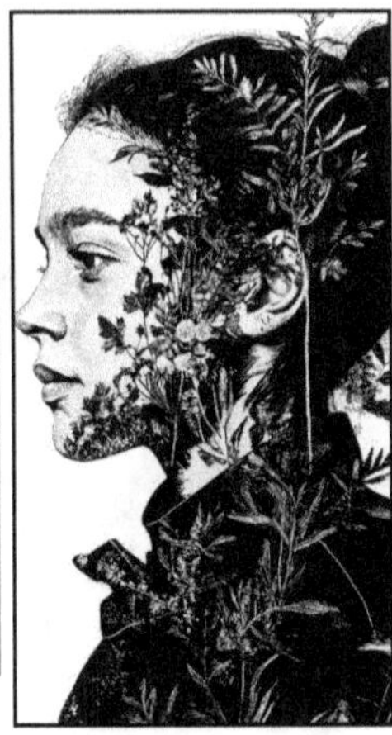 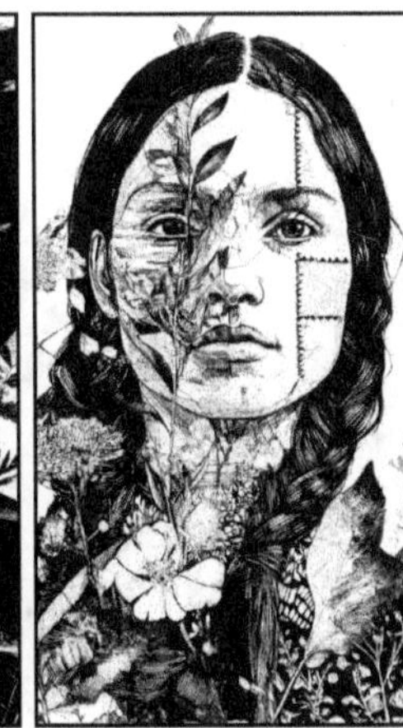 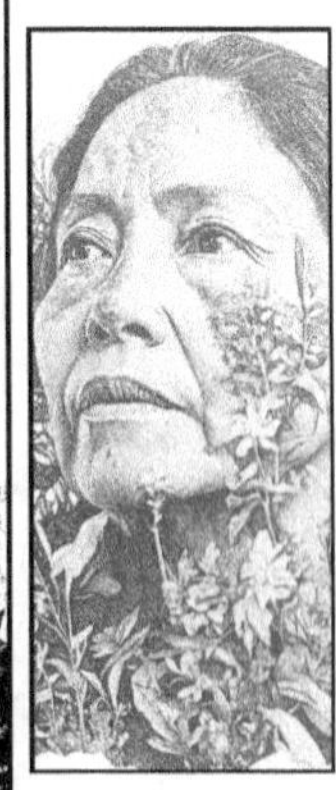

In North America, the perceptions and approaches to easing menstrual discomfort differ significantly between indigenous cultures and Western society. The ancestral customs of indigenous peoples are rooted in practices handed down from one generation to the next. In a time where medicinal plants take center stage, Eastern cultures embrace their healing power. Conversely, in Western societies like the United States and Canada, modern medicine holds sway, yet the allure of natural remedies and alternative therapies is on the rise.

The Rite of Isnati Awicalowanpi among the Oglalas

The Isnati Awicalowanpi ceremony is a sacred tradition of the Oglala people, a branch of the Lakota tribe, celebrating the transition into womanhood for young girls during their first menstruation. Firmly grounded in Lakota heritage, this ceremonial event is predominantly held on the Pine Ridge Reservation in South Dakota (United States) and is observed by various Sioux nations. While specific elements may differ from one family to another, this ritual endures as a powerful emblem of cultural strength amidst challenges of assimilation. Witness the beauty of its unfolding.

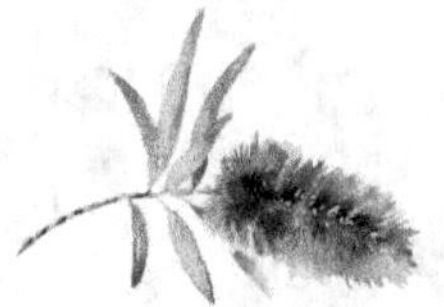

When the girl experiences her initial period, she is guided to a teepee located beyond the village. This revered area serves as a sanctuary for knowledge and contemplation, where she stays for multiple days.

A wise elder imparts wisdom about the duties that lie ahead as a future spouse and mother. These teachings encompass skills in managing a household, community involvement, and the spiritual essence of femininity in line with Lakota beliefs.

After the period of isolation, a special ceremony takes place, guided by a shaman. It aims to bestow blessings upon the girl, secure her future fertility, and mark her transition into the adult community. Through songs, prayers, and offerings, the spirits and ancestors are called upon for their protective presence.

Warm Sage Pouches

Warm pouches filled with sage leaves embody the traditional knowledge of Indigenous communities in North America, rooted in a deep connection with nature and its benefits. Sage (Salvia spp.), a sacred plant in many Indigenous cultures, is more than just a physical remedy; it is also a tool for spiritual and emotional healing.

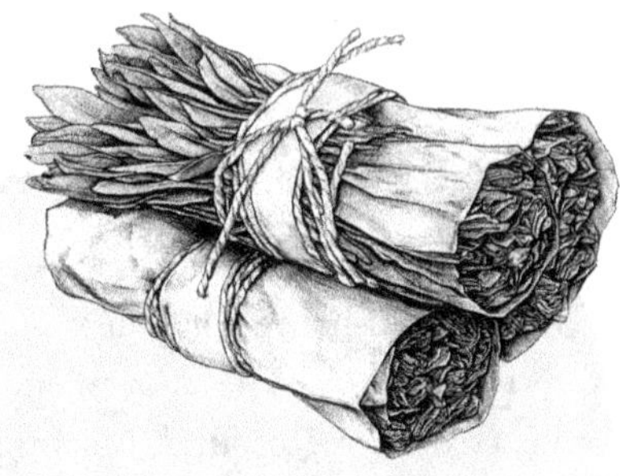

A COMPLETE THERAPEUTIC RITUAL

Heated pouches are much more than a simple method for relieving pain. Their use often fits within a broader framework of healing rituals, where the body and mind are treated as one. These rituals may include:

- A **moment of reflection** before applying the pouch, to establish a spiritual connection with nature.
- The **use of songs or prayers**, reinforcing the intention of healing.
- An **environment purified** with sage smoke (smudging), creating a sacred space for relaxation and care.

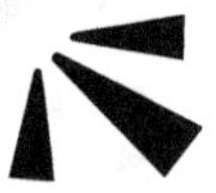

Yoga

Originating in India, yoga has garnered considerable attention in the Western world, especially in the United States and Canada, where it is seamlessly integrated into well-being routines. More than just enhancing flexibility, it provides substantial relief from menstrual discomfort by easing pelvic muscles, decreasing spasms, and enhancing blood flow. The accompanying breathing methods further aid in stress reduction, contributing to the alleviation of these discomforts.

POSE OF THE CHILD - BALASANA

- **Step 1 :** Begin in a kneeling position on the ground, gently separating your knees while ensuring your big toes remain touching.
- **Step 2 :** Embrace the movement by bowing down until your forehead connects with the ground, reaching your arms forward or resting them by your sides with palms upturned. Let go of any tension as you gently rest on your thighs, allowing your hips to find comfort over your heels. Inhale serenely, staying in this posture for as much time as you desire, soothing your lower back and releasing any stress.

POSE OF THE BUTTERFLY - BADDHA KONASANA

- **Step 1 :** Seated on the ground, extend your legs in front of you.
- **Step 2 :** Embrace the posture by bending your knees and uniting the soles of your feet, letting your knees open outward. Grasp your feet with your hands, then gracefully elongate your back. While maintaining a straight back, initiate leaning your upper body forward to your personal comfort level. Inhale deeply and sustain the position for a few minutes, elongating the muscles in your groin and hips, promoting relaxation in your pelvic region.

Natural Practices

In Western societies, women encounter growing health challenges magnified by the pressures of contemporary living. Persistent stress, poor nutrition, and rising sedentary habits all play a part in worsening various conditions, including those linked to menstrual discomfort.

Therapeutic heat offers a gentle and non-intrusive approach to alleviating menstrual cramps. By enhancing blood flow in the pelvic region, it aids in soothing the tense muscles of the uterus, thereby reducing discomfort efficiently.

Heating pads, hot water bottles, and heat patches are commonly embraced to offer instant relief, empowering women to alleviate their discomfort naturally and efficiently.

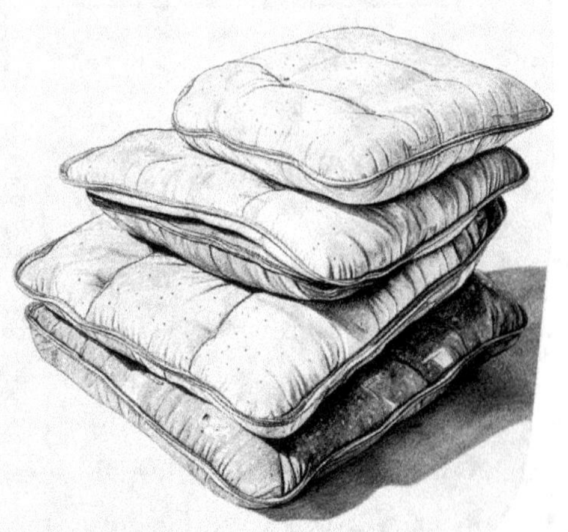

Central America

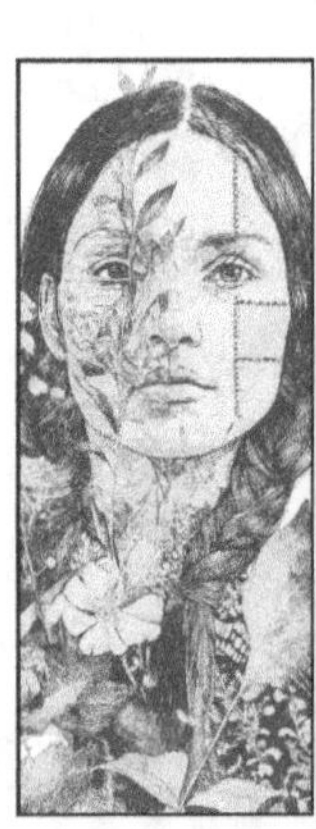 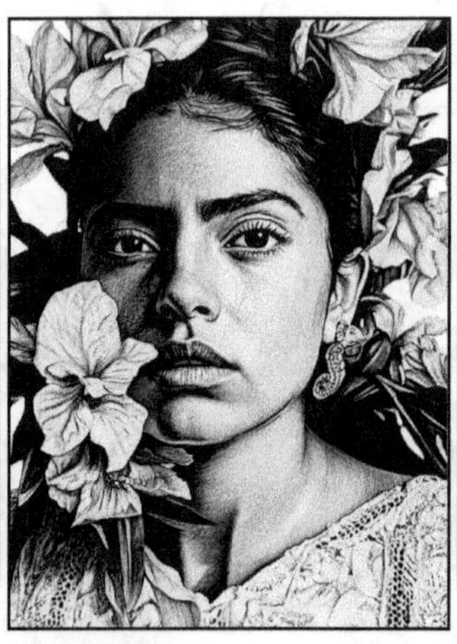 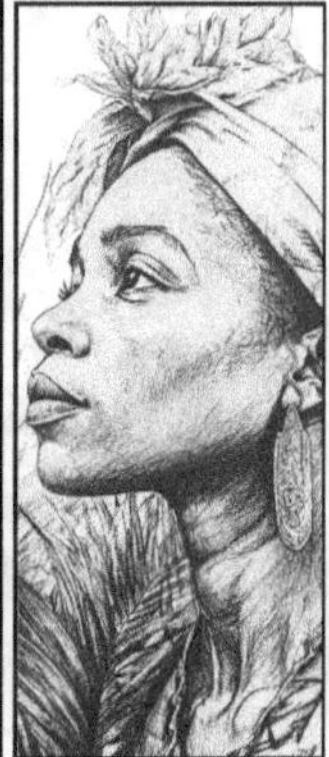 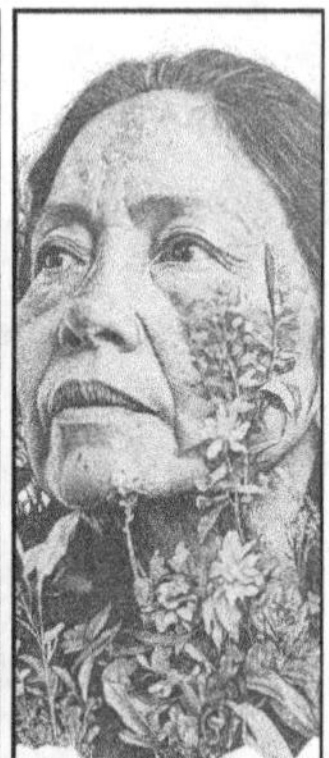 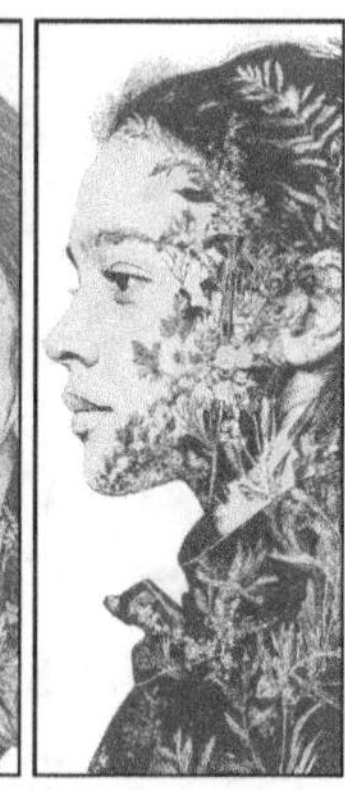

Central America, the birthplace of ancient civilizations like the Mayans and the Aztecs, holds a wealth of ancestral wisdom intertwined with a profound connection to nature. These communities have cultivated extraordinary expertise in healing plants, a legacy that is deeply ingrained. Still today, the women of this region carry on these traditions, utilizing herbal remedies to alleviate common ailments like menstrual pain, thereby safeguarding a valuable legacy amidst the trials of modernity.

The Sobadoras, Healers from Mexico

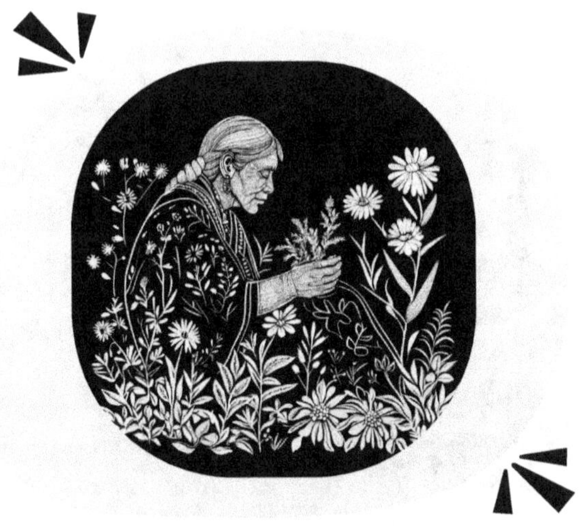

Sobadoras embody the essence of traditional healing, mastering the art of sobada. They hold a pivotal position in the realm of traditional healthcare in Mexico, especially in remote regions where modern healthcare services may be scarce.

Experienced women, the sobadoras have honed their skills through intergenerational transmission, often within their families. Their expertise goes beyond massage; they possess a deep understanding of medicinal plants, oils, and holistic healing methods. Along with addressing menstrual cramps, they apply their craft to various conditions like uterine repositioning, digestive problems, and postpartum discomfort.

The bond between the sobadora and her patients radiates trust and respect. Sobadoras embody wisdom within their community, offering more than just physical healing; they offer emotional and spiritual guidance, nurturing the complete well-being of those they care for.

Sobadora, Traditional Mexican Massage

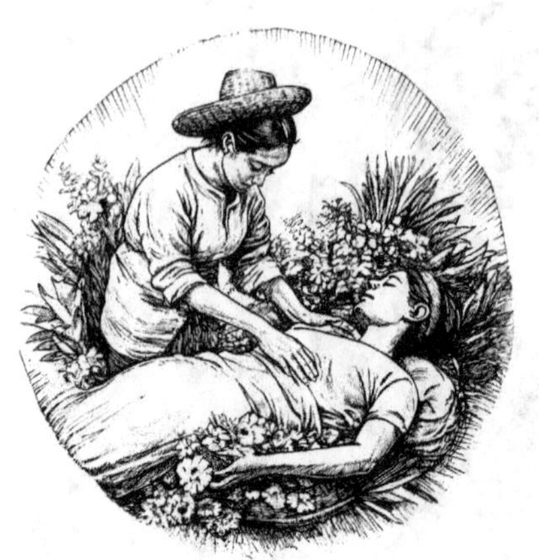

Sobada embodies a centuries-old Mexican practice, where skilled practitioners offer relief from menstrual discomfort. Through delicate circular motions, this massage incorporates arnica or castor oil known for their calming and anti-inflammatory qualities. By gently warming the oil in their hands, it enhances absorption and induces a tranquil state.

Following the massage, a chamomile infusion, known as **manzanilla**, is often suggested to extend the advantages of the treatment. Chamomile aids in alleviating stress and pain due to its soothing characteristics. This tradition, deeply ingrained in Mexican culture, holds significant importance in rural regions by providing both physical and emotional nourishment.

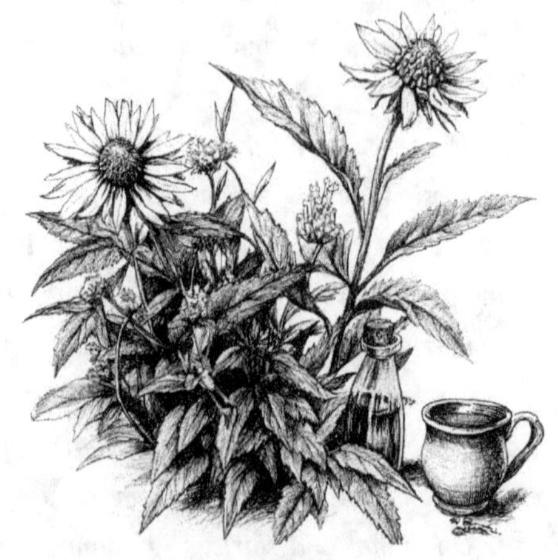

The Caribbean

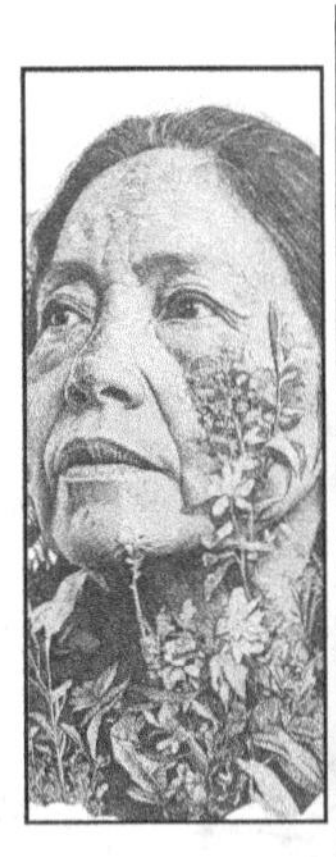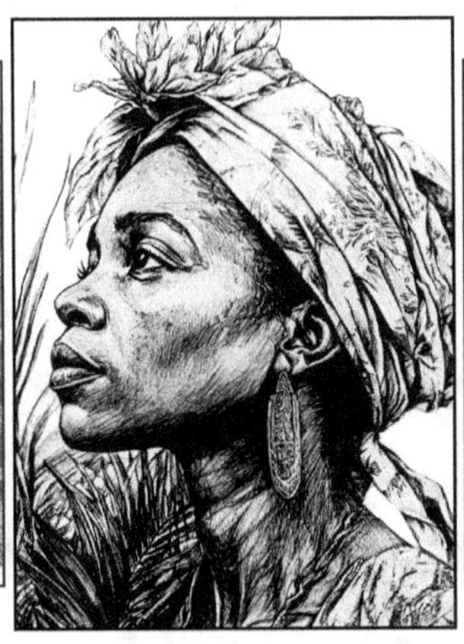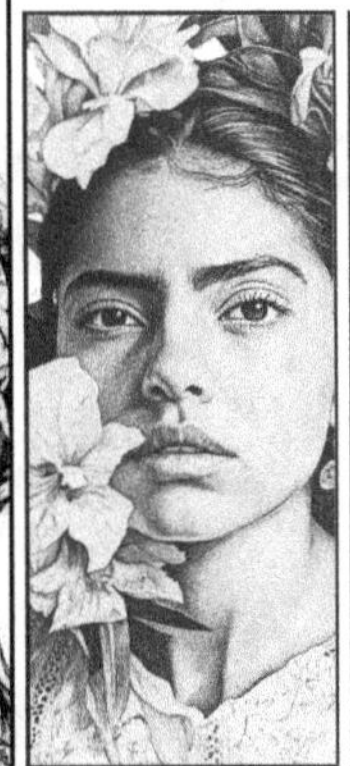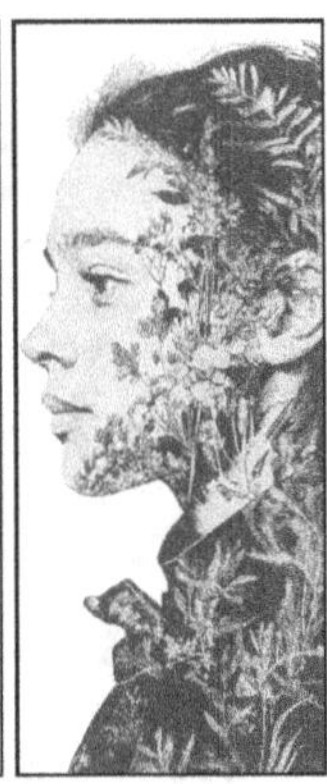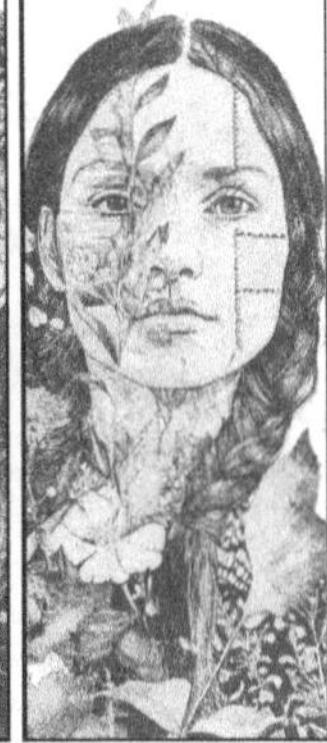

The Caribbean, abundant in a diverse culture, nurtures ancient wisdom shaped by African, European, Amerindian, and Asian legacies. These age-old customs, focused on natural remedies, showcase strength amidst the region's turbulent past. Every treatment carries a legacy, embracing a living heritage that intertwines Native American beliefs with African traditions. Cultivating medicinal plants under the Caribbean sun to address common ailments, such as menstrual pain, showcase the resilience and flexibility of this wisdom in overcoming modern obstacles.

The Secrets of the Curanderas

Throughout the colonial era in Central America, during the 16th and 17th centuries, Curanderas, known as healers, played vital roles in indigenous and mestizo societies, holding deep wisdom about healing herbs. These wise women, utilizing natural remedies like nopal, agave, and rue to address different illnesses, commanded both reverence and awe.

Yet, their impact was viewed as a challenge by the European colonizers, who interpreted these customs as sorcery. Blamed for striking a deal with the dark forces, these females faced persecution, trials, and death. This suppression sought to eliminate cultural defiance and enforce the religious and medical dominance of the colonizers.

Today, even as the traditions of the curanderas persist, the remnants of this era of oppression linger in the communal memory of the area. These healers personified a timeless wisdom, deeply connected to the natural world, whose influence is still evident in conventional medical customs today, echoing the strength and determination of native cultures in the presence of past adversities.

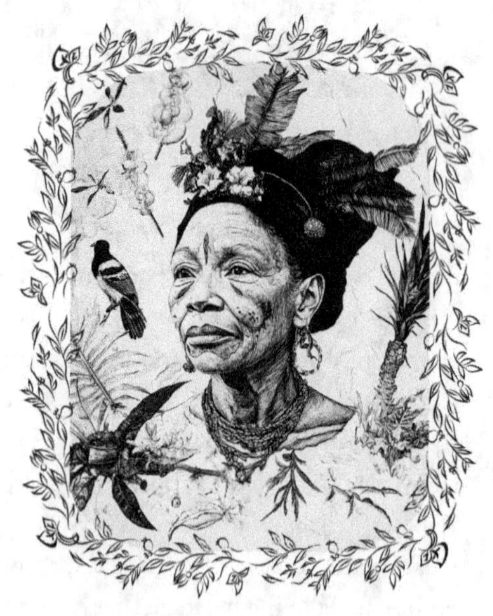

Plants

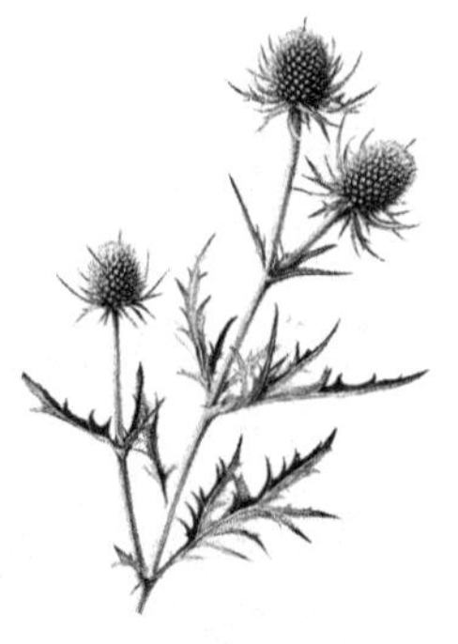

Referred to locally as **Chadon Beni** or **Culantro**, *Eryngium foetidum* is extensively utilized in Trinidad and Tobago and Grenada. Historically, its leaves are transformed into an infusion to alleviate menstrual cramps and other abdominal pains. Flourishing in damp, shaded regions, frequently found in Caribbean vegetable gardens.

Allspice, known as **Bois d'Inde**, thrives in Jamaica and Cuba. Its leaves and berries are brewed into infusions to ease menstrual cramps and abdominal discomfort. *Pimenta dioica* flourishes in tropical forests and well-drained soils, playing a vital part in local medicine and cuisine.

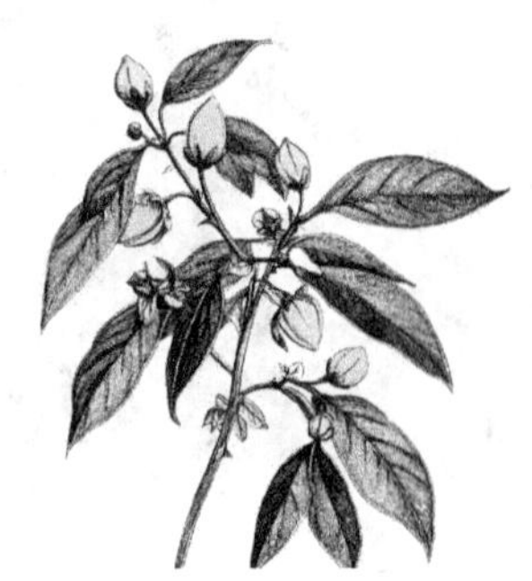

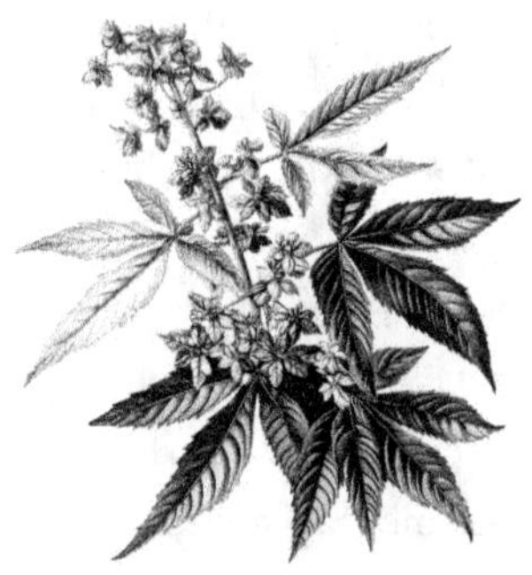

The **Castor bean**, discovered in various tropical areas, is grown and utilized in the Caribbean, notably in Jamaica. The oil derived from its seeds is frequently administered to the abdomen to alleviate menstrual cramps. Besides its topical application, **Ricinus communis oil** is at times consumed in small quantities for its gentle laxative properties, aiding in alleviating digestive unease linked to menstruation.

South America

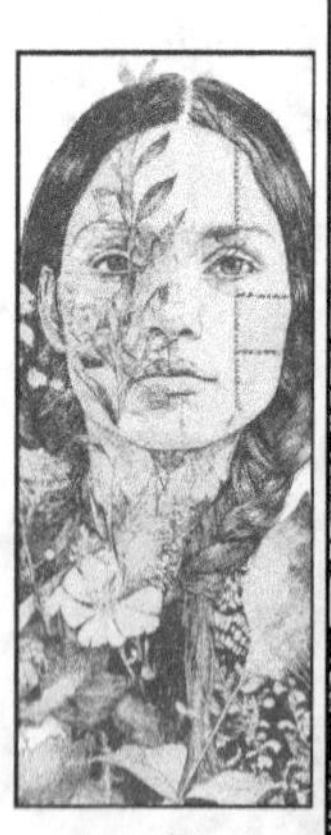
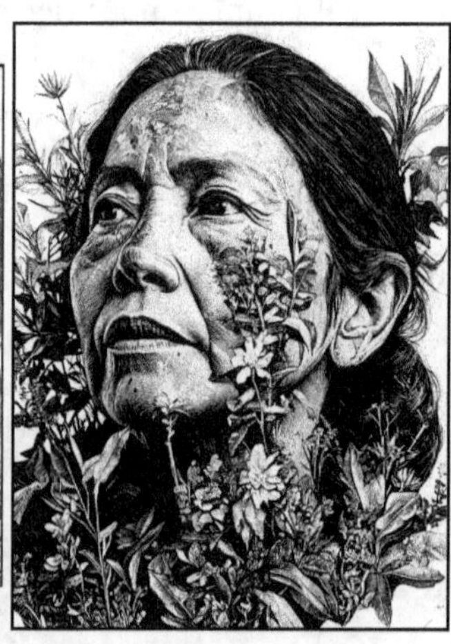
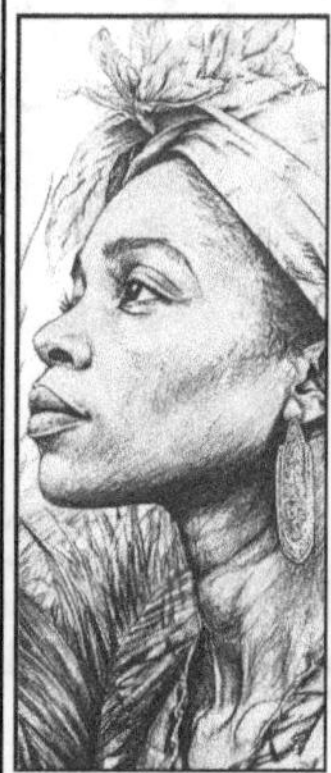
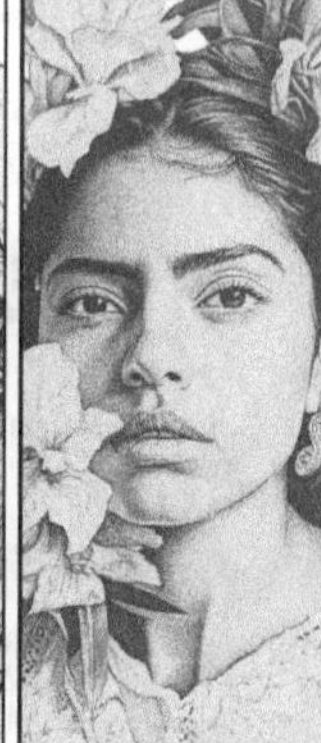
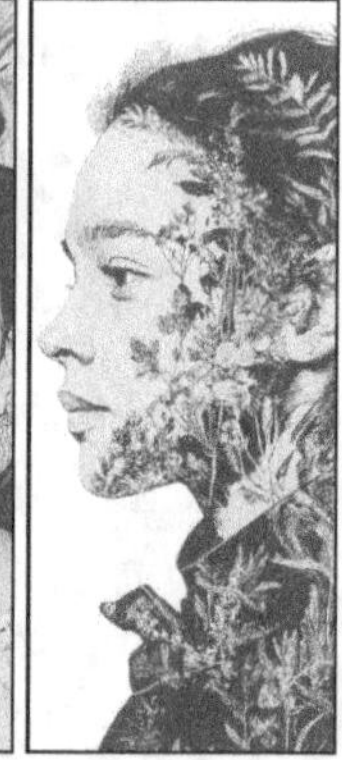

South America, abundant in contrasts and history, embodies a continent where ancient traditions persist due to women who safeguard and pass on wisdom concerning medicinal plants. Throughout the ages, in societies that hold nature in high esteem, these women have utilized indigenous plants. Local herbs like maca and coca leaf have been used for generations to alleviate different conditions, including menstrual discomfort. These traditions, deeply intertwined with symbolic and healing ceremonies, have endured through historical challenges and continue to be a fundamental aspect of health in numerous societies.

The Ticunas' Ceremonial Practices

The Ticunas embody the spirit of resilience and heritage. They dwell in the heart of the Amazon, tracing the winding path of the Amazon River through the lands of Brazil, Colombia, and Peru. Their ancient customs and profound wisdom have withstood the tests of time and external influences. Through a vibrant oral tradition, they pass down their stories, beliefs, and rituals from one generation to the next.

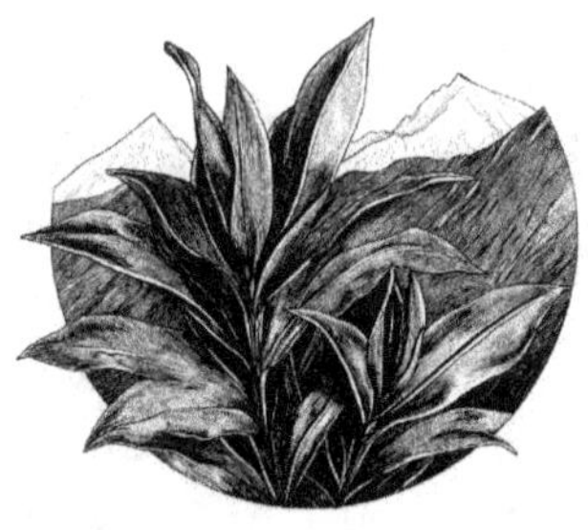

One of the most profound ceremonies in their culture involves the transition into womanhood for young girls, marking the beginning of their first menstruation. This pivotal journey commences with a phase of solitude, where young women step back from communal activities to immerse themselves in absorbing the wisdom and principles of their community. Throughout this period of self-reflection, they are mentored by the senior women, who educate them on ancestral stories, spiritual beliefs, and their roles within the community.

After the isolation period, a grand celebration is arranged to mark their return to the community and their transition into womanhood. This celebratory occasion serves as a tribute to their newfound maturity and a strengthening of the cultural bonds that bind the tribe together.

Maca Powder

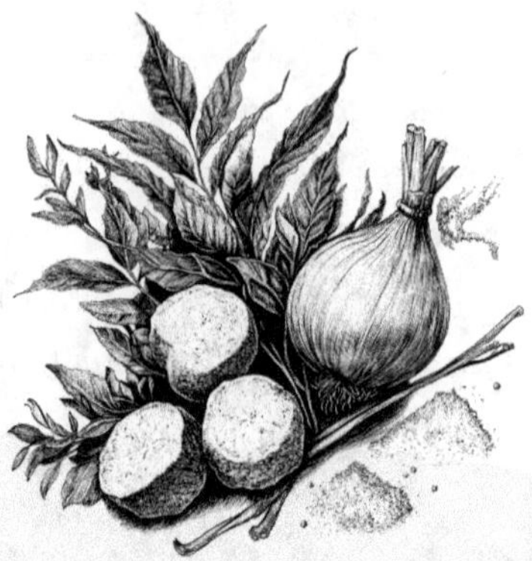

Maca, originating from the elevated lands of the Peruvian Andes, undergoes a traditional process of transformation into powder. Harvested when fully ripe, the Maca roots are sun-dried for days, occasionally even weeks, to decrease their moisture content. After achieving thorough dryness, the roots are finely ground into a powder, preserving all the plant's nutrients and medicinal qualities.

RECIPE

- Blend a teaspoon of maca powder into a glass of warm milk or hot water.
- Consume this elixir daily throughout menstruation to alleviate discomfort and harmonize hormones.

Maca enhances the menstrual cycle, alleviates menopausal symptoms, and boosts vitality.

Lorena's Seeds

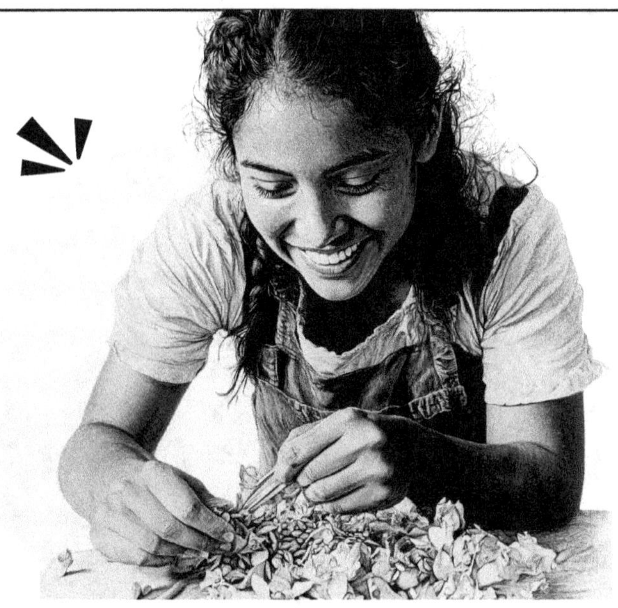

Lorena, deeply connected to her Colombian roots and a member of Vergers du Monde, shares precious knowledge rooted in the feminine traditions of her country: using seeds as natural allies to relieve menstrual pain and balance hormones. These practices draw on exceptional nutritional properties and simple techniques tailored to the specific phases of the menstrual cycle.

FOLLICULAR PHASE

(days 1 to 14 of the cycle)

LUTEAL PHASE

(days 15 to 28 of the cycle)

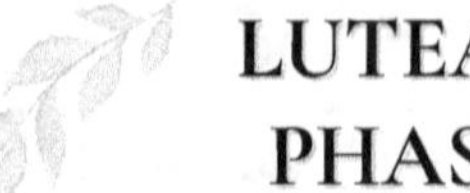

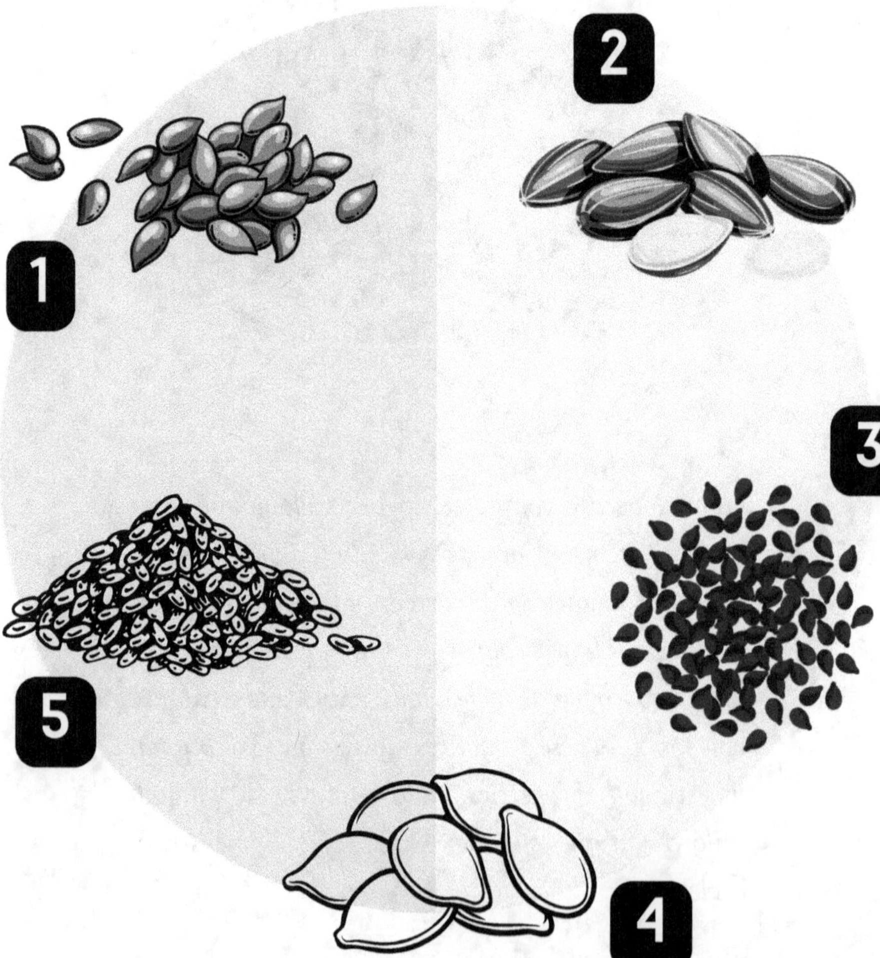

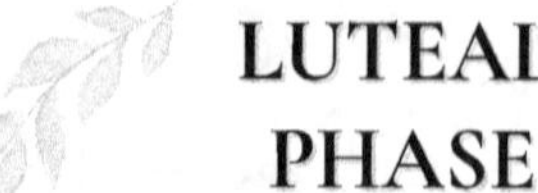

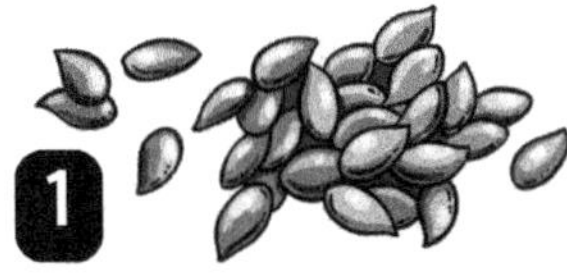

Flax Seeds: Rich in omega-3 fatty acids and lignans, they help balance hormone levels and can alleviate symptoms of premenstrual syndrome (PMS).

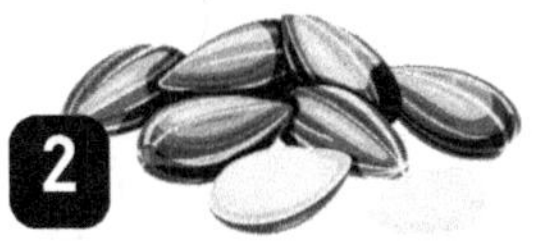

Sunflower Seeds: Contain zinc and magnesium, which are important for hormonal health and can reduce cramps and discomfort.

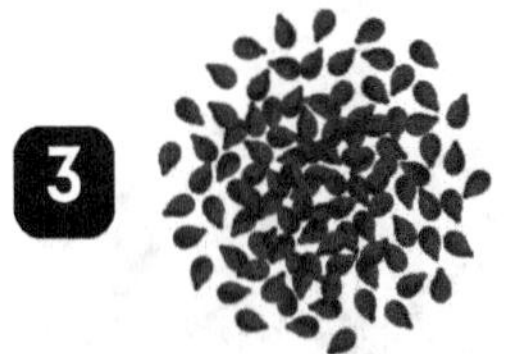

Sesame Seeds: A good source of calcium, which helps reduce menstrual pain.

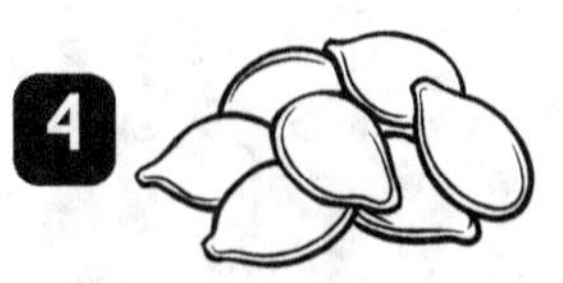

Pumpkin Seeds: Rich in zinc and magnesium, two essential nutrients for hormonal health, they help alleviate cramps and discomfort. They are also recommended for naturally boosting estrogen levels.

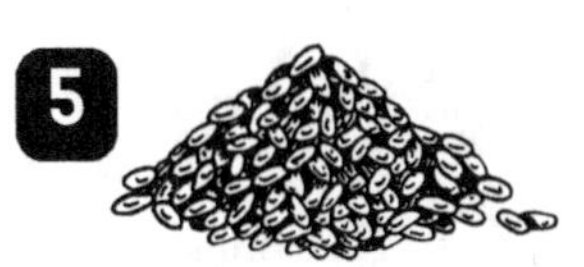

Chia Seeds: Packed with omega-3 fatty acids, they help balance hormones and reduce inflammation associated with PMS and menstrual cramps. They also support heart and brain health.

Recipes

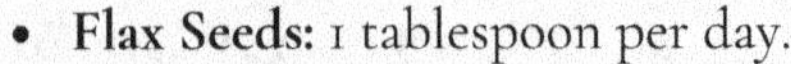

FOLLICULAR PHASE

- **Flax Seeds:** 1 tablespoon per day.
- **Pumpkin Seeds:** 1 tablespoon per day.

Both seeds can be consumed together, ground to facilitate nutrient absorption. These seeds promote estrogen balance during the first half of the cycle.

- **Chia Seeds:** 1 tablespoon per day.

They can be added to smoothies, yogurt, salads, soups, or cereals. Ideally, the seeds should be fresh.

LUTEAL PHASE

- **Sunflower Seeds:** 1 tablespoon per day.
- **Sesame Seeds:** 1 tablespoon per day.

These seeds support progesterone production. It is also preferable to consume them ground or crushed.

Tip: For flax and sesame seeds, consume them ground to enhance nutrient absorption.

Chia seeds swell upon contact with liquids, forming a gel-like texture. Soaking them in water, plant-based milk, or juice for at least 20 minutes before consuming makes them more digestible and allows nutrients to be better absorbed by the body.

CHAPTER 4
Oceania

POLYNESIA

AUSTRALIA

MELANESIA

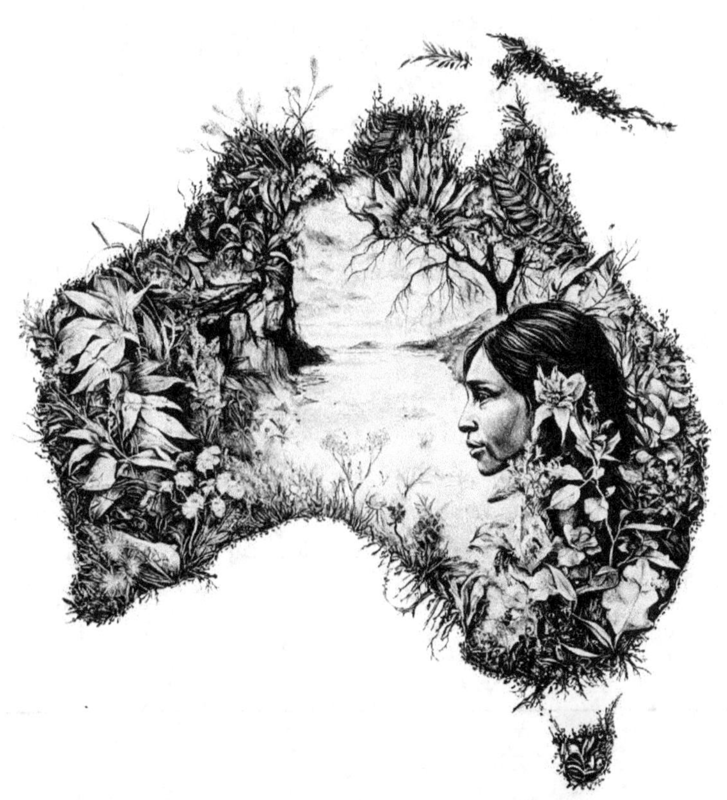

Polynesia

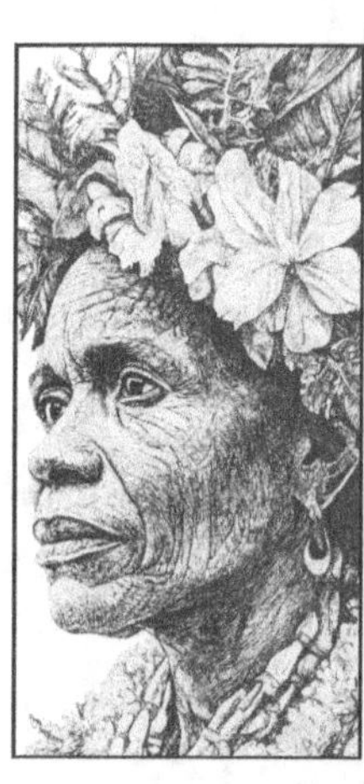
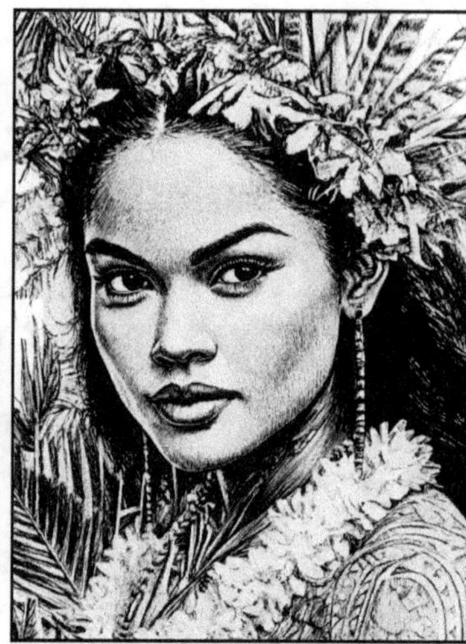
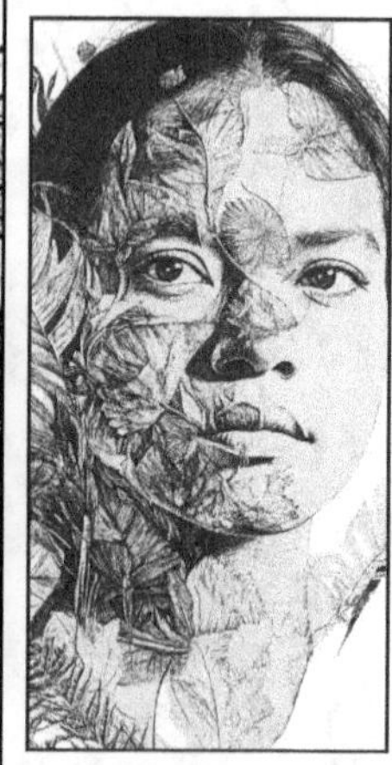

Polynesia, an extensive collection of islands spread across the Pacific, stands as a convergence of cultures molded by generations of island existence. Stemming from Austronesian migrations, Polynesian cultural communities like the Tahitians, Samoans, or Maoris have cultivated profound environmental wisdom.

In perfect harmony with their surroundings, traditional care practices, passed down from generation to generation, are deeply ingrained in daily life and mirror an intimate understanding of local plants and the sea that envelops them.

The Menstrual Cycle Guided by the Maramataka

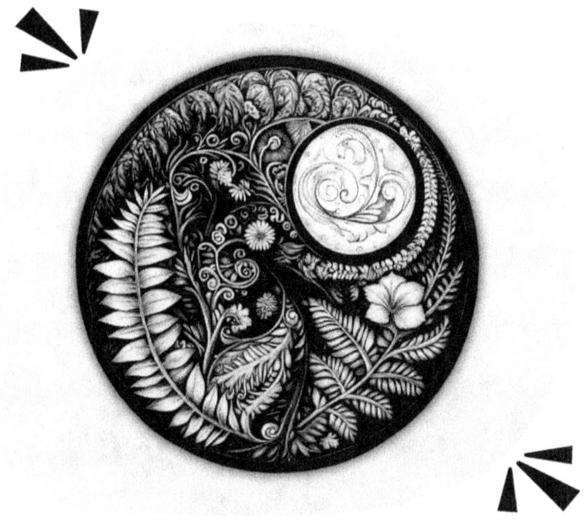

The Māori embody the heritage of New Zealand, a captivating island nation nestled in the southwest Pacific Ocean. Their presence graces the North Island (Te Ika-a-Māui) and the South Island (Te Waipounamu), where their culture flourishes, intertwined with the essence of the land and its abundant resources. Originating from Polynesia ages ago, the Māori have woven a tapestry of traditions that resonate through time.

Their traditional calendar, the **Maramataka**, serves as a guiding light for daily, agricultural, and spiritual endeavors. It goes beyond farming and fishing, intertwining with the body's natural rhythms, such as women's menstrual cycles. Specific moon phases hold significance for purification rituals, healing practices, and syncing with the female body's innate cycles. This integration weaves menstrual cycles into a broader tapestry of spiritual and physical existence.

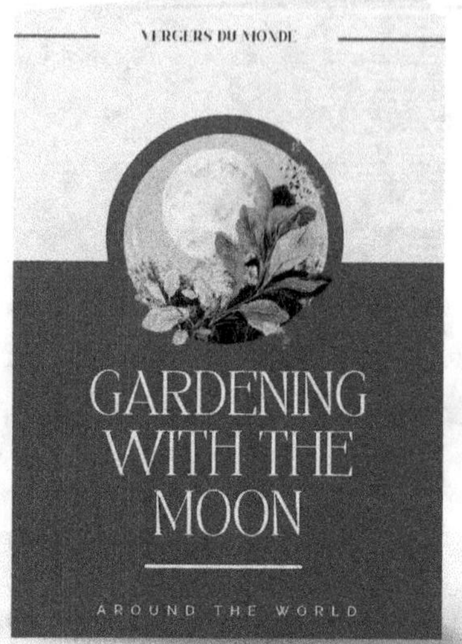

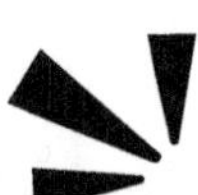

If the Maori culture and the impact of lunar cycles captivate you, make sure to explore our book **Gardening with the Moon around the World: Ancestral Farming Knowledge.**

This enchanting guide delves deeply into Maramataka and lunar influences, taking you on a voyage to the core of these ancestral traditions. A essential read for nature enthusiasts and seekers of ancient wisdom!

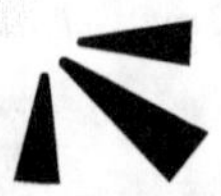

Noni and Miri Leaf Elixir

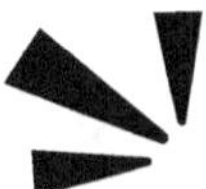

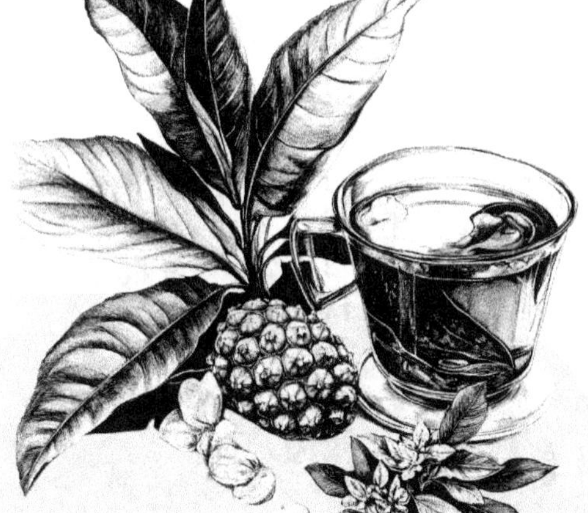

INGREDIENTS

- Noni foliage (Morinda citrifolia)
- Miri Leaves (Glochidion ramiflorum)
- Hot water

PREPARATION

- Boil a handful of noni and miri leaves in water for approximately 10 to 15 minutes.
- Allow the infusion to cool down gently and strain it.
- Consume this herbal infusion twice daily throughout your menstrual cycle to calm discomfort and harmonize the body's energies.

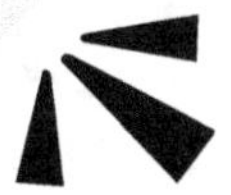

Australia

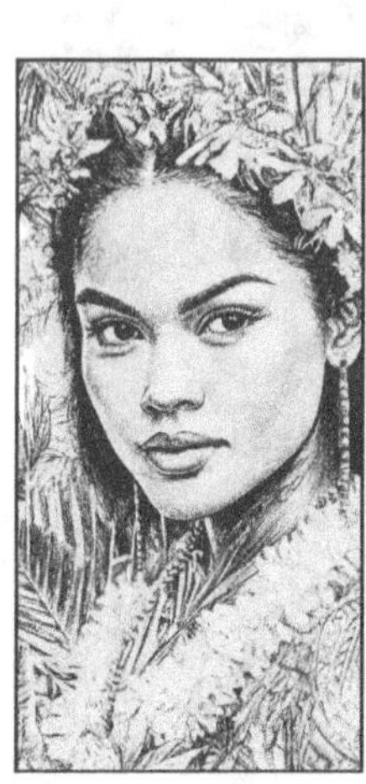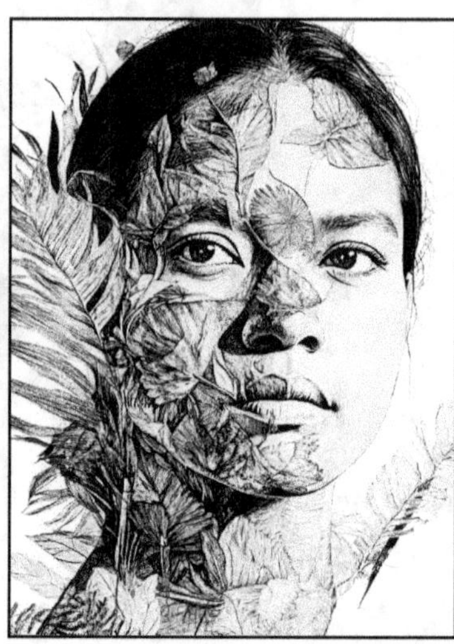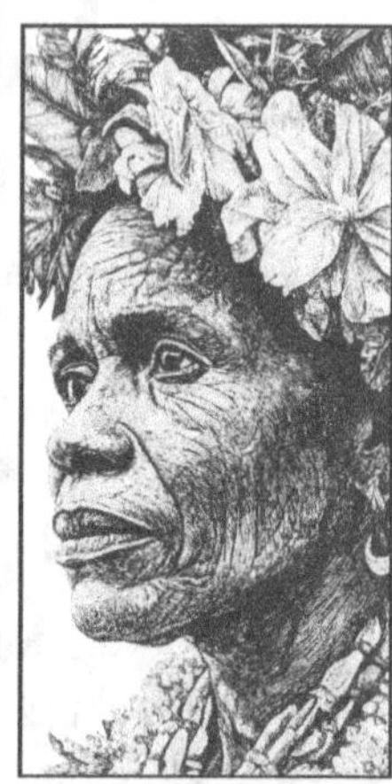

Australia, a land of vast wilderness, is home to one of the oldest cultures globally: that of the Aborigines. For thousands of years, these first inhabitants have developed ancestral wisdom in deep harmony with their surroundings, where each plant and each ritual is infused with spiritual significance.

The Aborigines honor the land as a vibrant being, commemorating the Dreamtime, a legendary era when forefathers molded the earth. Nowadays, these crucial and age-old customs face challenges from modernity, yet endure due to the strength of a community that upholds their rituals and heritage.

Bush Medicine

Rooted in the age-old traditions of the Australian Aborigines and the peoples of the Torres Strait, **Bush Medicine** is based on the use of native flora and fauna for physical and spiritual healing. The healers of these communities, true guardians of this ancestral knowledge, play a crucial role in maintaining the health of their people. The Aborigines have developed a deep knowledge of the medicinal properties of local plants, whether to treat illnesses or to accompany rites of passage.

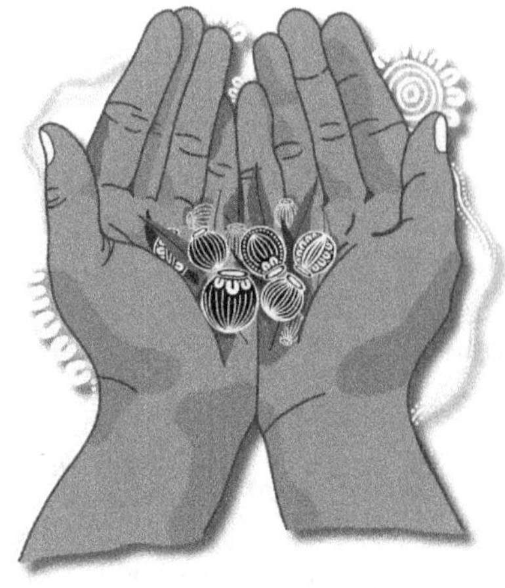

Certain Aboriginal communities observe secretive and respectful passage ceremonies for young girls, known only within their community. Rituals like **Djunba** and **Wongga**, although more documented for other purposes, are linked to female initiation rites in some communities. These sacred ceremonies signify the journey of young girls into womanhood and are typically led by female elders who impart crucial wisdom for their upcoming lives.

Ngurunderi, another term linked to Aboriginal folklore and ceremonies, embodies a range of tales and customs connected to creation and ancestral spirits. The intricate aspects of these rituals, especially those concerning young girls, are seldom disclosed openly because of their confidential essence. This confidentiality highlights the cultural and spiritual significance of these traditions, designed to safeguard and enlighten young girls on their life journey.

Goanna Tree Decoction

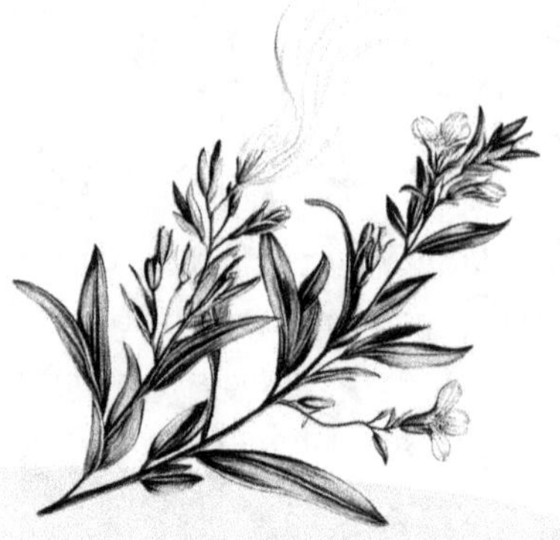

*The **Goanna Tree** holds great value for its soothing impact and anti-inflammatory characteristics. Indigenous communities view it as a potent solution for alleviating various types of pain, such as menstrual cramps.*

- The Goanna tree's leaves are frequently gathered and brewed to create a decoction. This remedy is utilized both internally, as a beverage to alleviate internal discomfort, and externally, administered to injuries to encourage recovery.

- The tree's bark plays a significant role in ancient customs. It can be burned, and the resulting smoke is utilized in cleansing ceremonies or to calm restless souls. This tradition is frequently associated with sacred gatherings, with the purpose of purifying either the surroundings or the individuals involved.

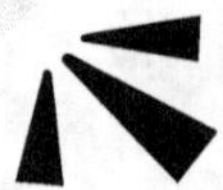

Melanesia

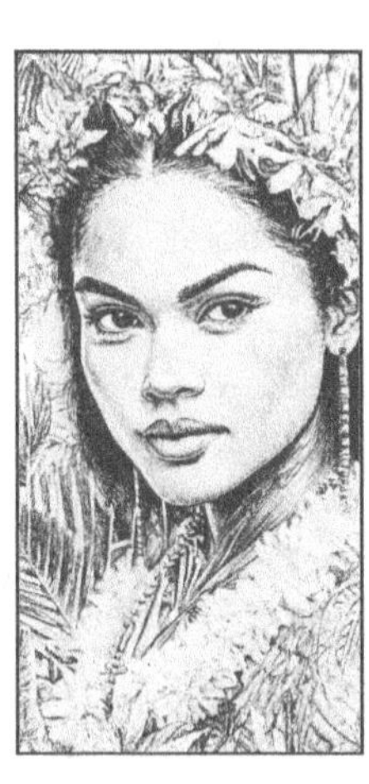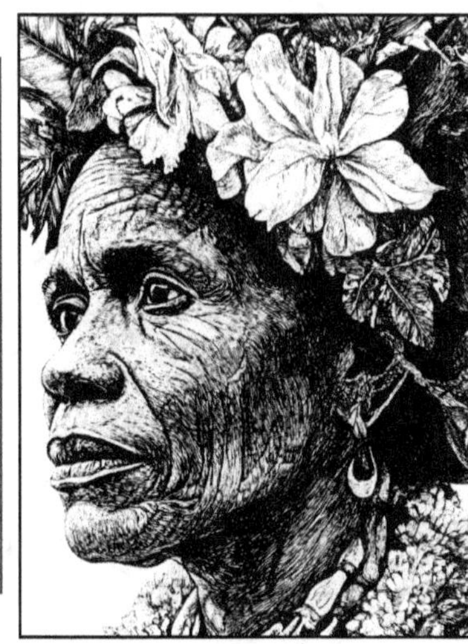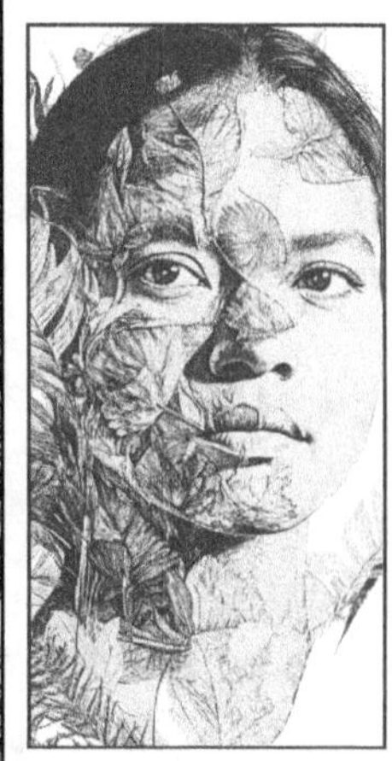

Melanesia, situated in the southwest Pacific, encompasses archipelagos like Papua New Guinea, the Solomon Islands, Vanuatu, and New Caledonia. The area is distinguished by remarkable ethnic diversity, boasting hundreds of unique languages and cultures. Women in Melanesia hold a pivotal position in the passing on of wisdom.

Ancient wisdom, especially in healthcare, is deeply woven into the fabric of Melanesian societies. The adept utilization of indigenous plants to heal various illnesses seamlessly weaves ancestral insights into everyday existence. These customs harmonize with communal life and the ceremonies that adorn Melanesian cultures.

Mama Graun

*The Melanesian islands are home to a diverse tapestry of tribes, each embracing unique languages, traditions, and ancient healing wisdom. Within these communities, healers, known as **mama loas** or **mama graun**, embody a crucial presence. Predominantly women, these revered individuals possess profound expertise in herbal remedies and sacred ceremonies. They stand as the cornerstone of ancestral healthcare, especially for women.*

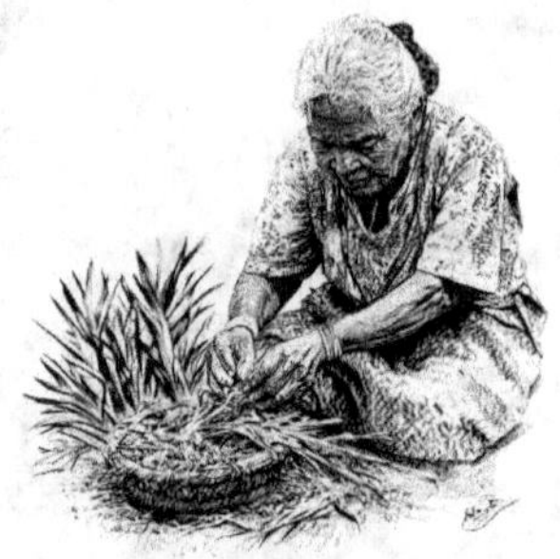

On the island of Tanna in the Vanuatu archipelago, healers share a deep connection with the land and natural rhythms. Their healing methods go beyond basic remedies; they encompass rituals for fertility, coming-of-age ceremonies for young women, and specialized care for women's health during menstruation and childbirth. Mama loas, in particular, harness the power of indigenous plants to create natural remedies for easing menstrual discomfort and supporting the birthing process. In Papua New Guinea, the rich tapestry of tribes like the Huli, Asaro, or Tolai, manifests in the array of healing plants and rituals. The mama graun in these villages hold a vital position in guiding young girls into their femininity, imparting wisdom on plant remedies and the significance of nature's rhythms. These lessons, typically transmitted from one generation to the next, are infused with reverence for the earth and forebears.

Plants

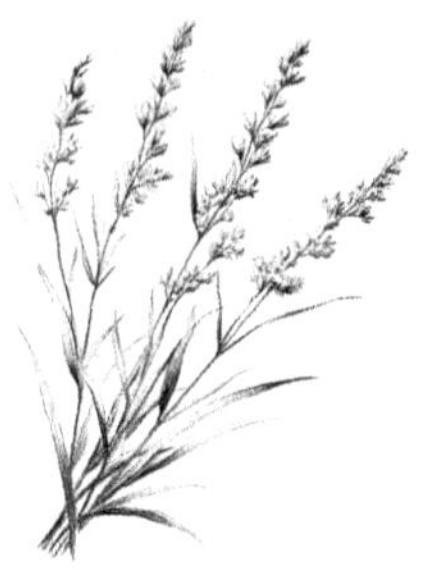

Eleusine indica, also called *hiroi* or *iquazi* in various regions of Papua New Guinea, is a bountiful herb flourishing in open or disturbed spaces like roadsides and lawns. The leaves and stems of Eleusine indica are brewed into a decoction to alleviate menstrual issues. This elixir is believed to harmonize the menstrual cycle and alleviate related discomfort.

The *Hibiscus rosa-sinensis*, known locally as b*anban (Hisiu)* or *hibiscus (Waiwa)*, is a shrub belonging to the Malvaceae family. A brew made from the young flower shoots is utilized to alleviate menstrual discomfort and balance the cycle. Additionally, pregnant women are offered flowers and leaves soaked in coconut juice to stimulate labor.

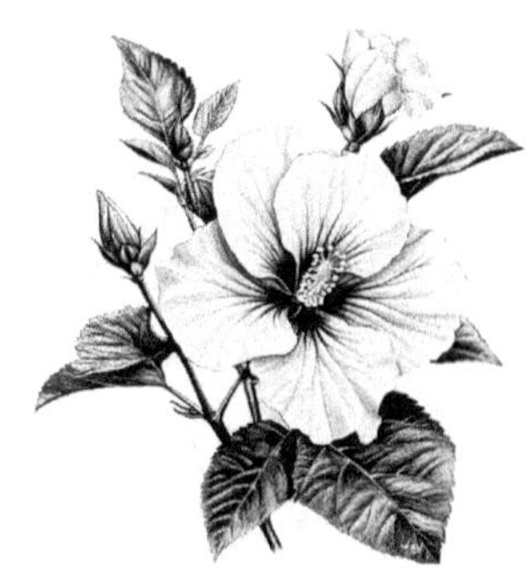

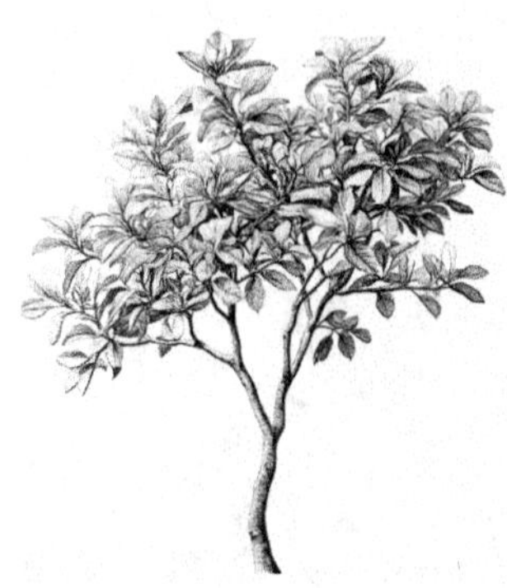

Homalanthus novoguineensis, known locally as *ngohou (Kurti)* and *hikumutu (Siwai)*, is a shrub or tree that can reach heights of ten meters, commonly found in secondary forests. Despite its toxic nature, this plant has been traditionally utilized to address a variety of ailments: its warm young leaves are employed in abdominal massages. A unique practice linked to menstruation involves consuming a mixture of sap and water for three days, known for its potent contraceptive properties and ability to induce menstruation.

CHAPTER 5
Europe

EASTERN EUROPE

WESTERN EUROPE

MEDITERRANEAN EUROPE

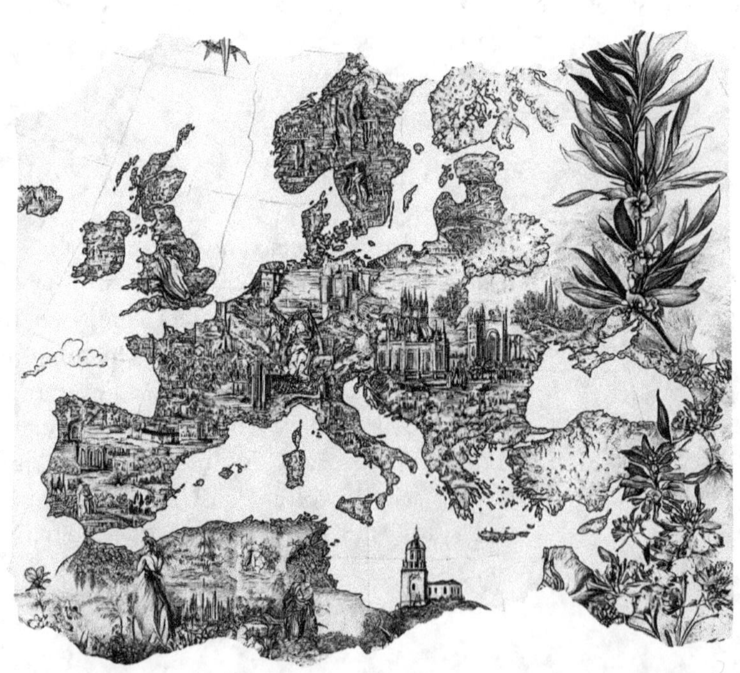

Eastern Europe

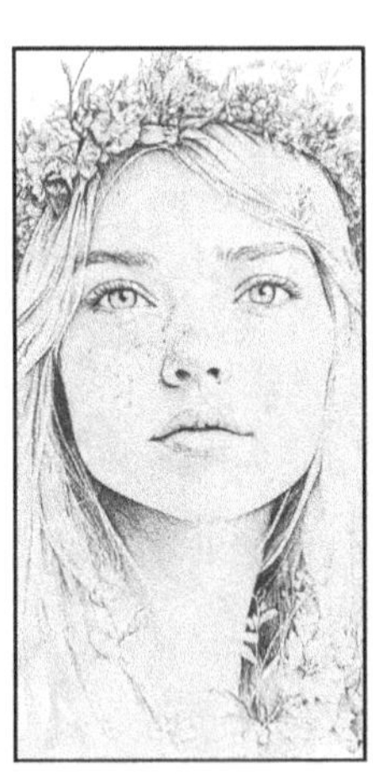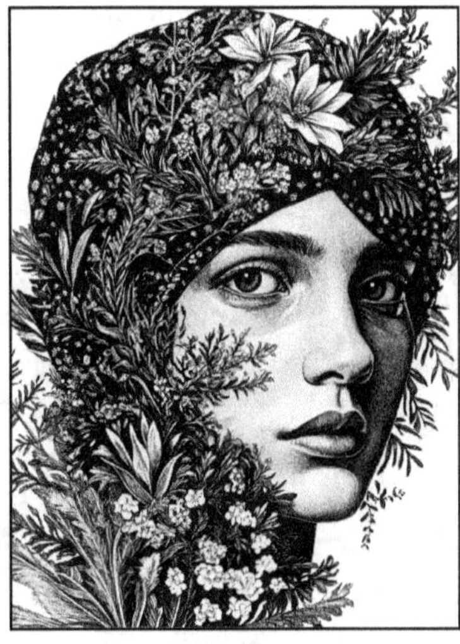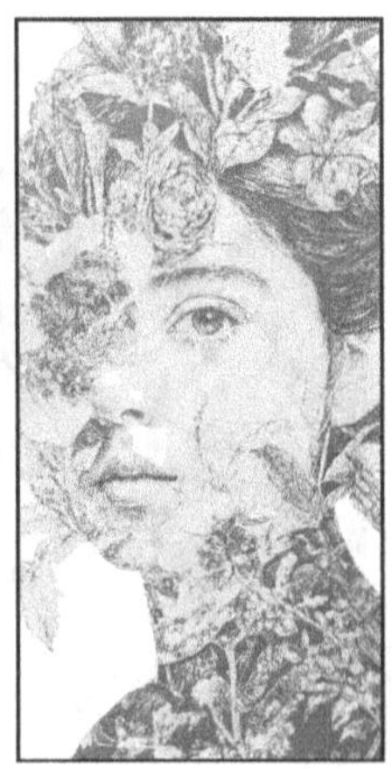

Eastern Europe, a vast expanse extending from the Carpathians to the Russian plains, is characterized by a tapestry of ancient cultures and traditions. This land, shaped by a rich history of empires and nomadic tribes, holds an immeasurable treasure trove of folk wisdom. Women often hold the key, their wisdom intertwined with nature, unveiling ancient secrets where nearby plants transform into valuable companions in everyday rituals.

Banya, Russian Steam Bath

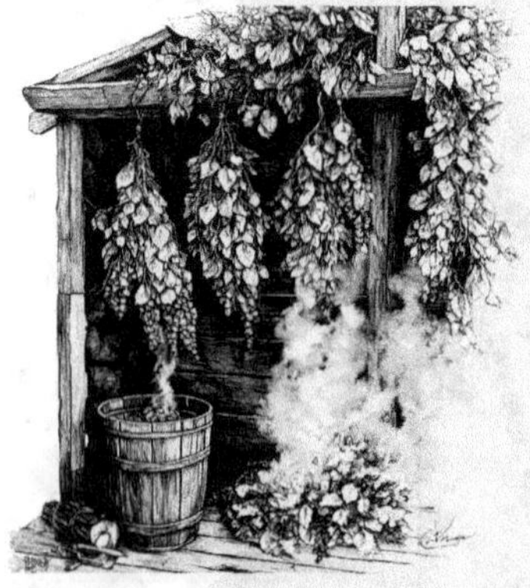

The ***banya (баня)***, a ritual from Russian culture, traces its origins back to ancient times, long before the Christian era in Russia. Inherited from the Slavic peoples, this tradition has endured through the centuries, maintaining its pivotal role in daily life. Initially, the banya served not just hygienic functions but also spiritual ones, being viewed as a sanctuary for purifying the body and soul.

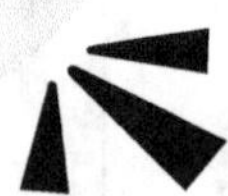

The banya journey entails embracing the warm humidity, reaching temperatures near one hundred degrees Celsius, to unlock the pores, purify the skin, and enhance blood flow. Central to this practice is the utilization of the ***venik (веник)*** – a cluster of dried twigs, typically ***birch (берёза)*** or ***oak (дуб)***, to gently strike the body. This action not only boosts blood circulation but also induces muscle relaxation and skin renewal.

The powerful warmth aids in calming the abdominal and pelvic muscles. The banya, enveloped in its comforting and cleansing ambiance, transforms into a sanctuary where women can reestablish a bond with their bodies and alleviate the discomforts associated with their menstrual cycle.

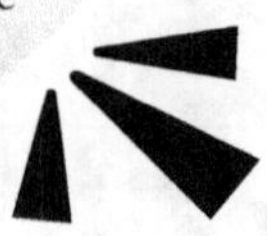

Plants

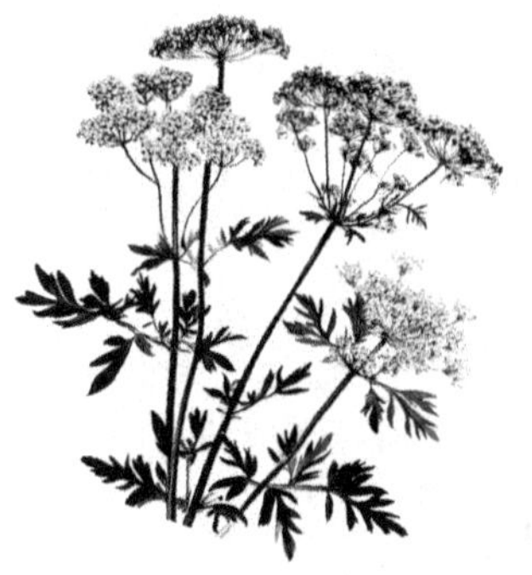

Yarrow (Achillea millefolium), known as *Coada-șoricelului* in Romanian, is widely embraced throughout the Balkans. Celebrated for its antispasmodic qualities, this plant is a beloved remedy often brewed into a comforting herbal tea to ease menstrual cramps. The dried flowers are carefully infused for this purpose. Flourishing in meadows and sun-kissed spots, this plant is cherished for its innate potency.

Rowan (Sorbus aucuparia) - known as *Jarząb* pospolity in Polish, thrives as a tree across Eastern Europe. The vibrant red berries, packed with antioxidants, are commonly dried and brewed to alleviate menstrual cramps. Drawing from Polish heritage, this uncomplicated solution brings natural relief.

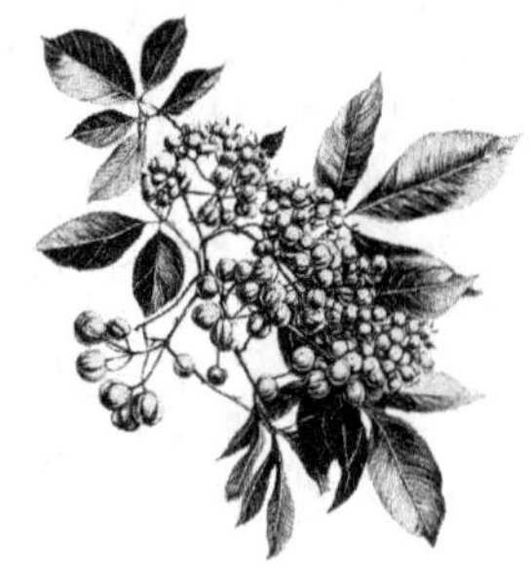

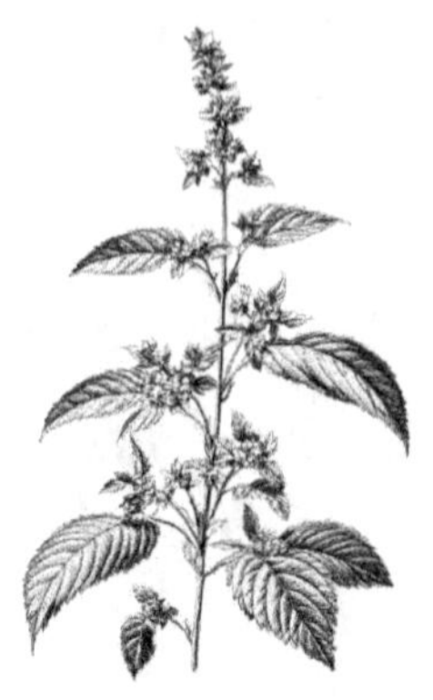

Known as *Žihľava* in Slovak, *Nettle (Urtica dioica)* is also valued in Romania, Poland, and Hungary for alleviating menstrual cramps. Abundant in iron and minerals, it is frequently enjoyed as a soothing herbal infusion. By steeping the dried leaves in boiling water for ten minutes, a beneficial tea is created. Flourishing in damp, shaded locations, nettle is celebrated for its anti-inflammatory and strengthening qualities, making it a perfect aid for easing menstrual discomfort.

Western Europe

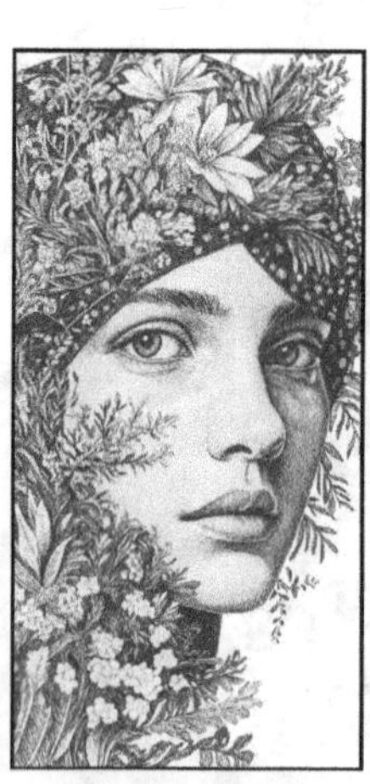
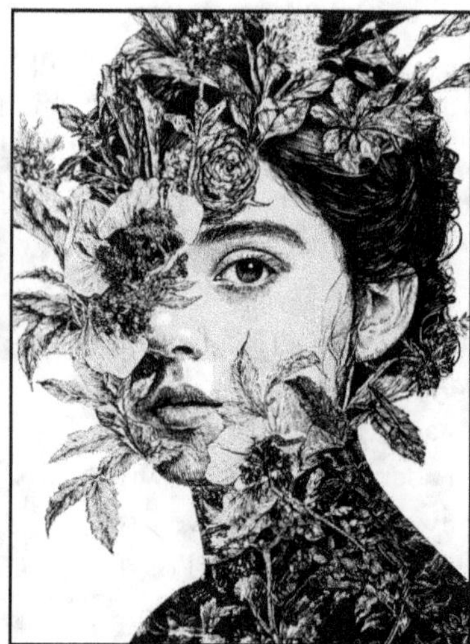
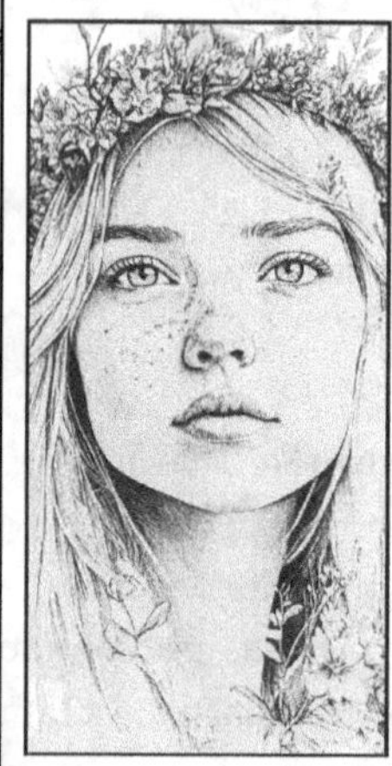

Western Europe, encompassing nations like France, Germany, the United Kingdom, Spain, and Italy, stands as a timeless continent defined by a deep history and diverse cultural impacts. As the birthplace of numerous civilizations, it has experienced significant social transformations, especially during the industrial revolution led to the loss of much traditional knowledge. Today, with a renewed interest in natural medicine, these ancestral practices are experiencing a renaissance, while Western societies seek to find a balance between modernity and well-being.

Aromatherapy

Aromatherapy, a practice with roots dating back to ancient civilizations like Egypt, Greece, and Rome, has made a comeback in the daily routines of Western Europeans. This revival is driven by an increasing longing to utilize natural and holistic approaches to address different ailments, such as menstrual cramps, showing a preference for nature-based remedies over solely chemical treatments.

Aromatherapy involves utilizing essential oils, derived from fragrant plants, for their healing qualities. Each oil possesses distinct properties, spanning from relaxation to boosting the immune system, including alleviation of menstrual discomfort.

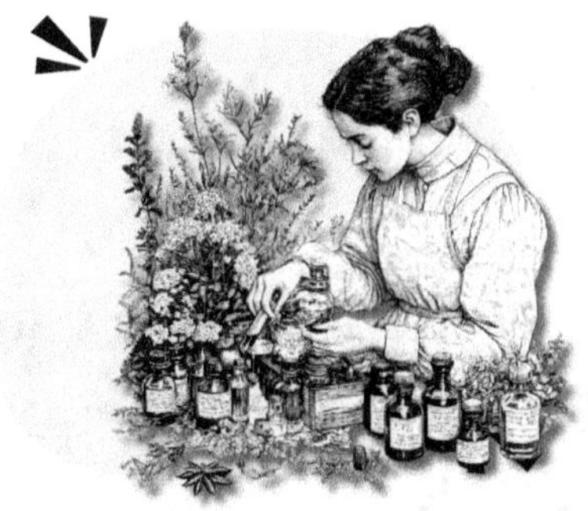

France houses numerous experts in aromatherapy and cultivators of herbs, benefiting from a rich history of perfumery and herbal medicine. In contrast, the United Kingdom, although thriving in this area, embraces a broader approach to herbal medicine, incorporating essential oils into comprehensive therapies.

Essential Oil of Lavender

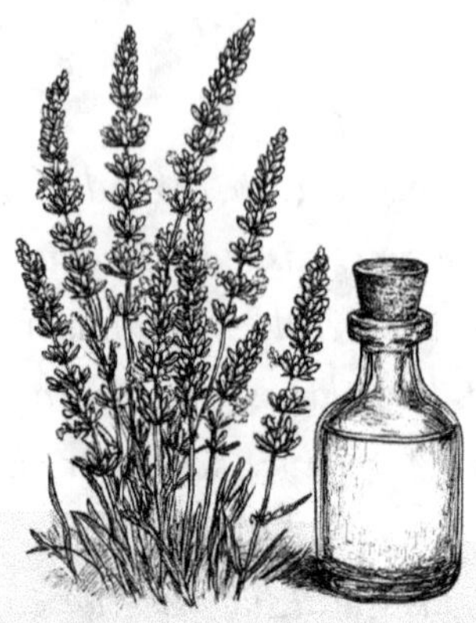

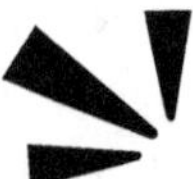

Lavender essential oil, derived from **Lavandula angustifolia**, renowned for its calming qualities, aids in relaxing abdominal muscles and alleviating menstrual cramps.

INGREDIENTS

- A vial of lavender essential oil
- 1 tablespoon of nurturing vegetable oil (sweet almond or jojoba)

PREPARATION AND IMPLEMENTATION

1. Blend lavender essential oil with vegetable oil in a tiny bowl.
2. Apply the blend to the lower belly with soft circular motions for a couple of minutes.
3. Perform the application two to three times daily throughout the menstrual cycle to alleviate discomfort.

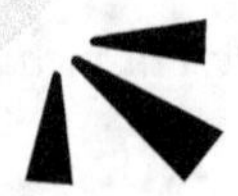

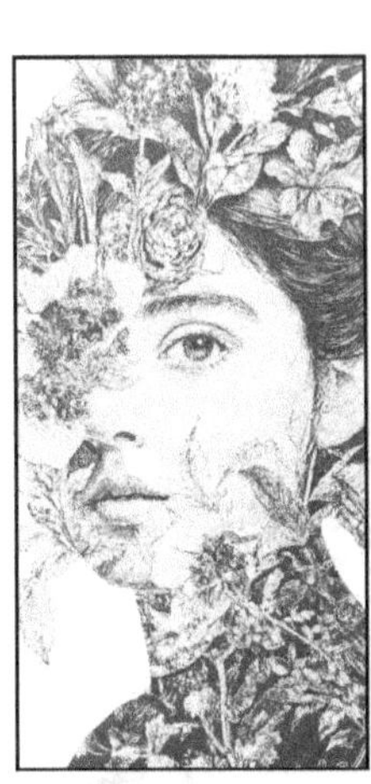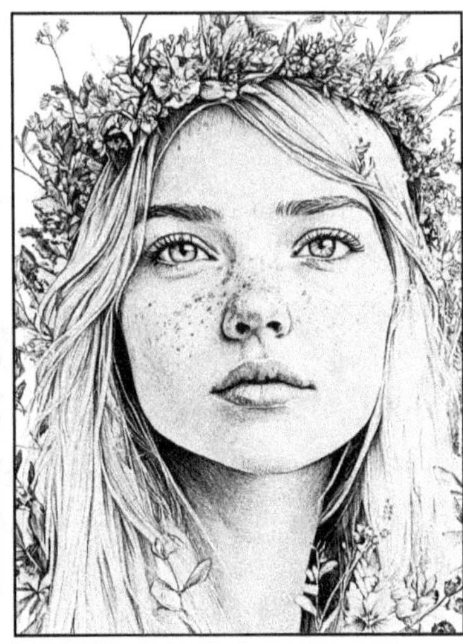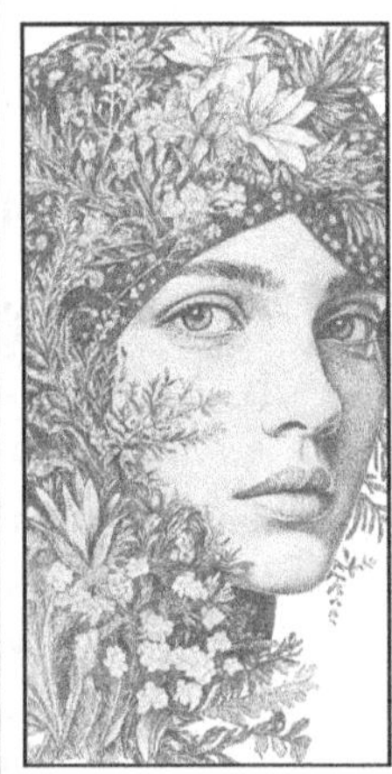

The Nordic countries, encompassing Sweden, Norway, Denmark, Finland, and Iceland, stand as beacons of social progress and well-being. However, the topic of periods, like in other places, remains veiled in secrecy and hush. Over the years, these nations have been dedicated to destigmatizing menstruation, blending art, politics, and social initiatives to dismantle biases. In societies that cherish equality and transparency, menstruation is starting to be acknowledged not just as a biological reality but also as a cultural and political matter.

Scandinavian Sphagnum Moss

In Scandinavia, up until the 20th century, *sphagnum moss* from peat bogs served as a vital absorbent. It was a key component in daily life, especially for menstrual protection and diapers, due to its rich absorbent qualities.

To harness its power, vibrant moss, whether white or red, must be gathered from undisturbed peat bogs and then meticulously dried before application.

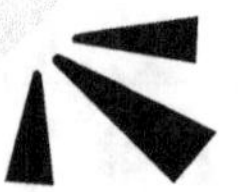

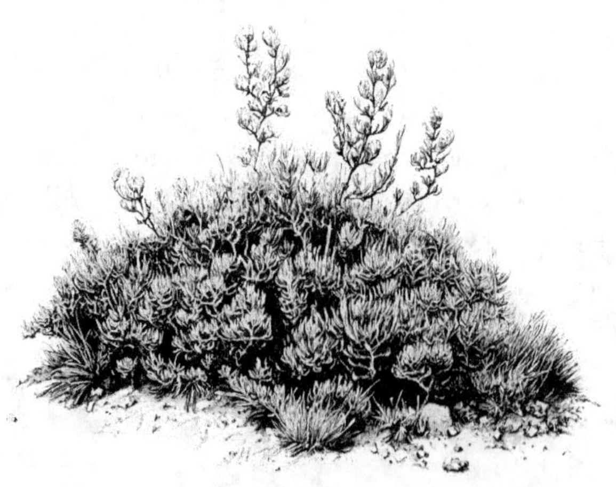

Juice of Berries

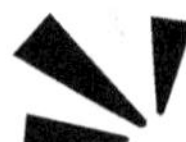

*Northern berry juices, such as **lingonberries**, **blueberries**, and **raspberries**, provide a delightful and effortless means to embrace their health advantages. Abundant in bioactive compounds, these fruits thrive in chilly environments, aiding in alleviating menstrual cramps and promoting holistic well-being.*

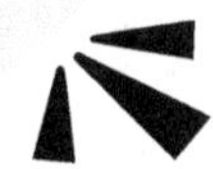

Lingonberries, blueberries, and raspberries flourish organically in boreal and temperate forests in northern regions. They prosper in infertile, acidic soils, frequently in shady undergrowth or forest clearings, where cool, moist conditions support their growth. Abundant in flavor and health advantages, lingonberry, blueberry, and raspberry juices are known for their anti-inflammatory and antioxidant properties. These juices are often used to soothe menstrual cramps and are essential for maintaining health, particularly in regions with limited access to fresh produce. By adding these juices to your daily diet, you can effortlessly harness the power of these natural remedies.

CHAPTER 6
Middle East

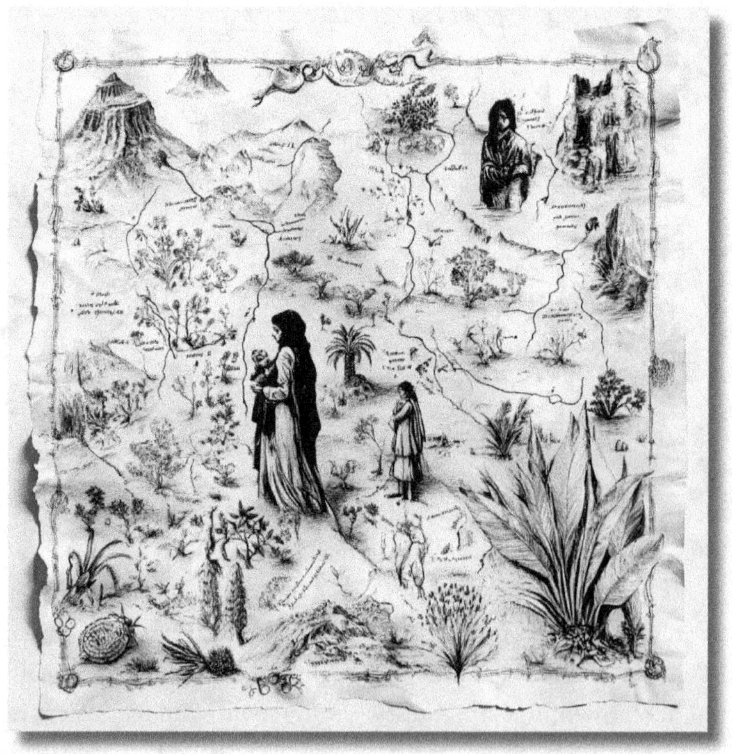

ARABIAN PENINSULA

PERSIA AND MEDITERRANEAN

LEVANT DESERT

Arabian Peninsula

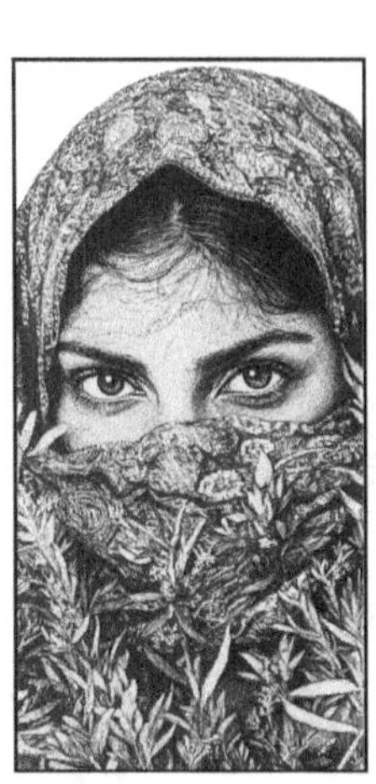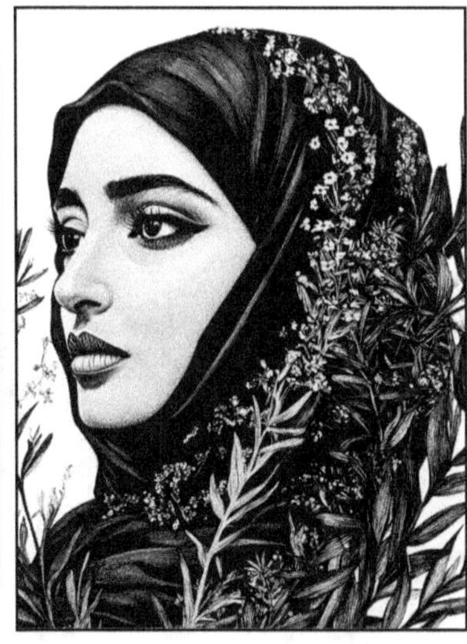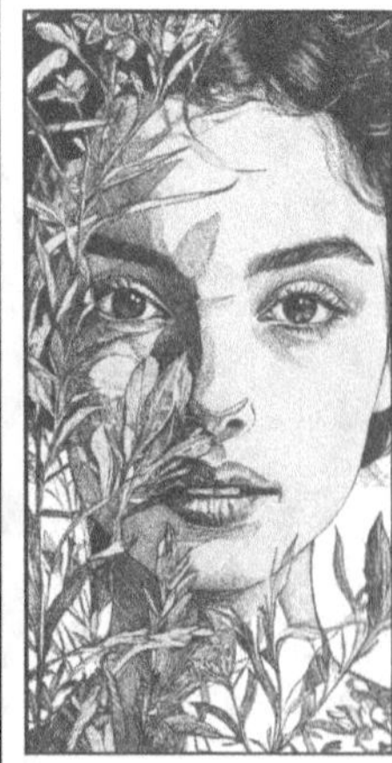

The Arabian Peninsula, encompassing Saudi Arabia, the United Arab Emirates, Oman, and Yemen, holds a treasure trove of healing wisdom handed down through ages. These time-honored customs, intertwined with indigenous traditions, blend ancestral remedies with local rituals, and emphasizing the utilization of indigenous flora, valuable resins, and fruits, each contributing significantly to sustaining the health and vitality of communities. These natural treatments, deeply rooted in daily existence, persist in mirroring a vibrant and invaluable cultural legacy.

Traditions

The **Tibb an-Nabawi** embodies ancient wisdom on health and well-being, encompassing guidance on hygiene, nutrition, and the benefits of natural remedies like **black seed (Nigella sativa)** for various health issues.

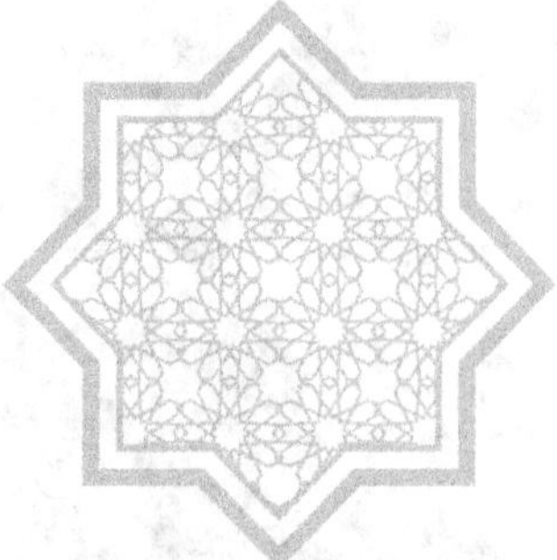

The enduring reverence and application of these age-old treatments persist today, particularly in the rural regions of the Arabian Peninsula, where access to contemporary healthcare may be limited.

Incorporating plants and resins, these customs encompass rituals like **hijama (cupping)** and herbal infusions, aimed at cleansing the body and addressing different health issues, including menstrual disorders. These practices are frequently combined with prayers and invocations, strengthening the link between physical well-being and spirituality.

Passed down from generation to generation, these remedies continue to hold a central place in the daily lives of the Arabian Peninsula residents, embodying a harmonious blend of ancestral wisdom and spiritual traditions.

Resinous Plants

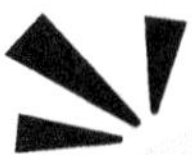

Myrrh, recognized as مرّ *(Mur)* in Arabic *(Commiphora myrrha)*, emerges from the dry lands of the Arabian Peninsula. Celebrated for ages for its healing and cleansing qualities, it is often brewed into a comforting infusion to alleviate menstrual discomfort. Myrrh can be gently spread as a paste or oil to ease inflammation and abdominal cramps.

Frankincense, known as لبان *(Luban)* in Arabic, emanates from the Boswellia sacra tree, flourishing predominantly in the dry terrains of the southern Arabian Peninsula, notably in Yemen, Oman, and Somalia. Esteemed for its anti-inflammatory and calming attributes, frankincense is commonly inhaled or administered as a balm to alleviate menstrual and joint discomfort. The process involves burning the resin for inhalation of the fragrant fumes or crafting a paste for direct skin application.

Persia and the Mediterranean

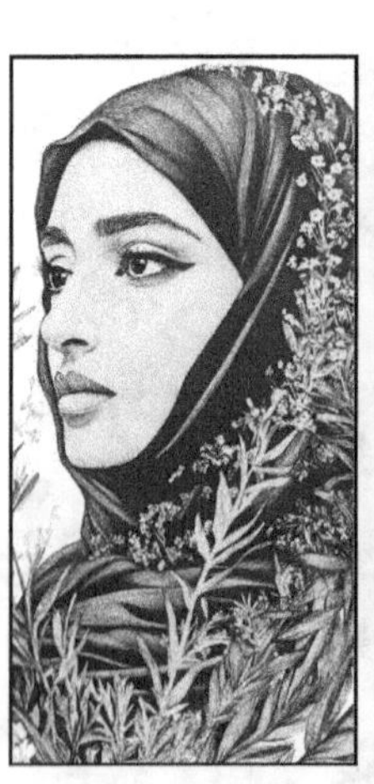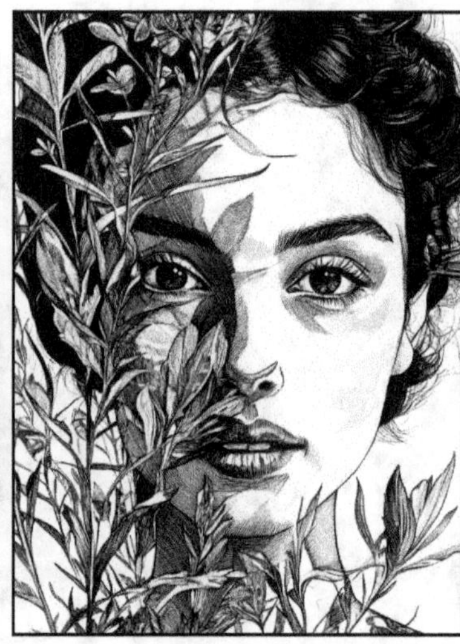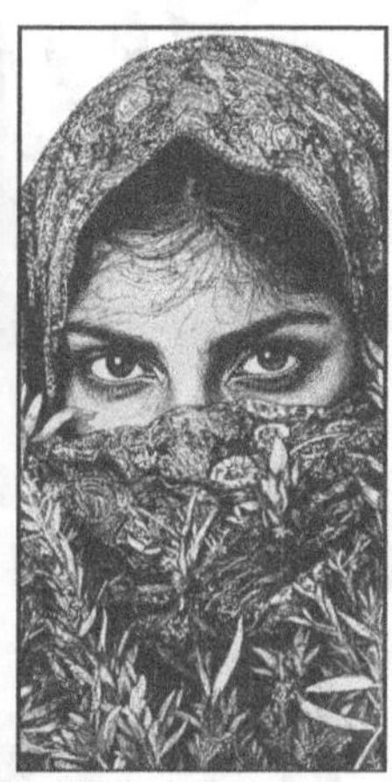

The Persian and Eastern Mediterranean region embodies a convergence of Roman, Greek, Persian, and Arab influences that have sculpted a civilization of extraordinary richness. This land, characterized by vast cultural diversity, serves as the birthplace of ancient traditions that have endured through the centuries.

Ancestral wisdom emerged there, thriving to expand far beyond their borders. The utilization of thyme, for instance, introduced by the Greeks, extended to Europe. From the Damascus rose to the sacred myrrh, these lands are a boundless spring of natural remedies, safeguarded and enhanced over the ages.

Plants

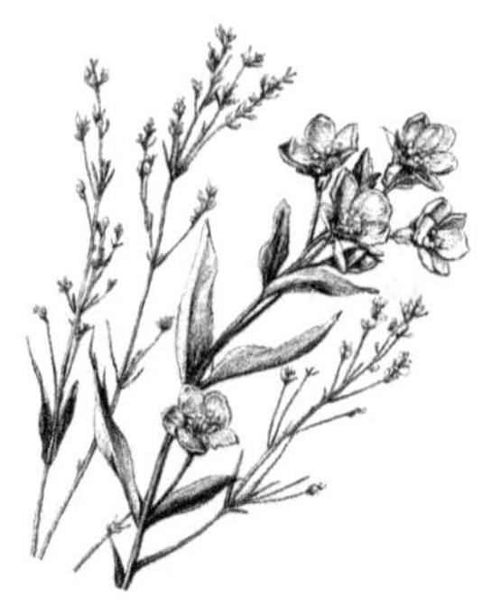

Rue (Ruta graveolens), also known as السذاب *(Al-Sadhab)* in Arabic, is a healing plant indigenous to the Mediterranean regions such as Iran, Lebanon, and Syria. Celebrated for its antispasmodic and emmenagogue qualities, rue has been utilized since ancient times. The leaves of rue are brewed into an infusion to alleviate menstrual discomfort and balance menstrual cycles, especially in the cultural practices of these areas.

Fenugreek, Trigonella foenum-graecum, or حلبة *(Helba)* in Arabic, is a plant widely grown in the Middle East. Consumed in decoction or infusion, fenugreek seeds are known to help ease menstrual discomfort and balance hormones, a popular remedy embraced by women in these areas.

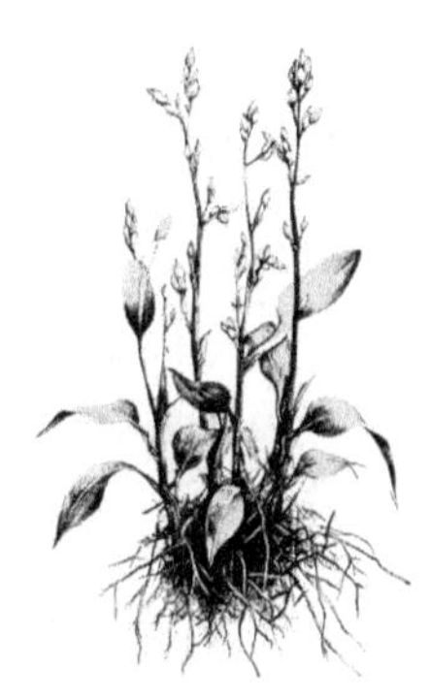

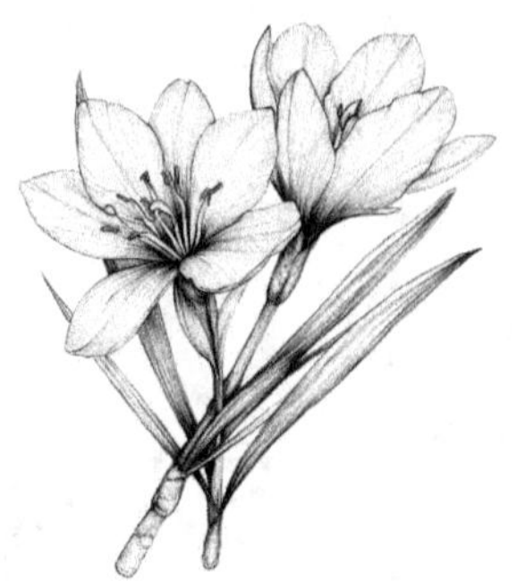

Saffron, also known as زعفران *(Za'fran)* in Arabic, is a valuable spice extracted from the stigmas of the crocus flower *(Crocus sativus)*. Originating from Iran, saffron is grown in various regions of the Middle East and the Eastern Mediterranean. Traditionally used as an infusion to ease menstrual discomfort, saffron's antispasmodic and calming qualities aid in reducing cramps and balancing menstrual cycles.

Water of Damask Rose

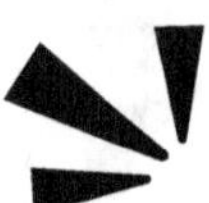

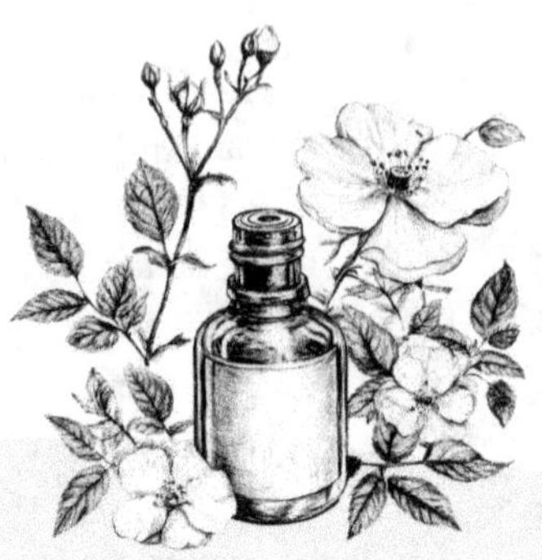

*Rosa damascena, or **Damask Rose**, holds a special place as one of the most precious and historic types of roses, highly cherished in Iran and the eastern Mediterranean regions. Its uses are diverse:*

FLORAL ELIXIR

Distilled from petals, rose water nourishes and calms the skin, serving in purification ceremonies and as a facial toner.

INFUSION

Steeping rose petals creates a fragrant tea with calming qualities, also helpful in soothing menstrual cramps and digestive issues.

VITAL ELIXIR

Rose essential oil, distilled for its renowned relaxing, aphrodisiac, and anti-inflammatory properties, is commonly used to alleviate muscle pain and tension.

Levant Desert

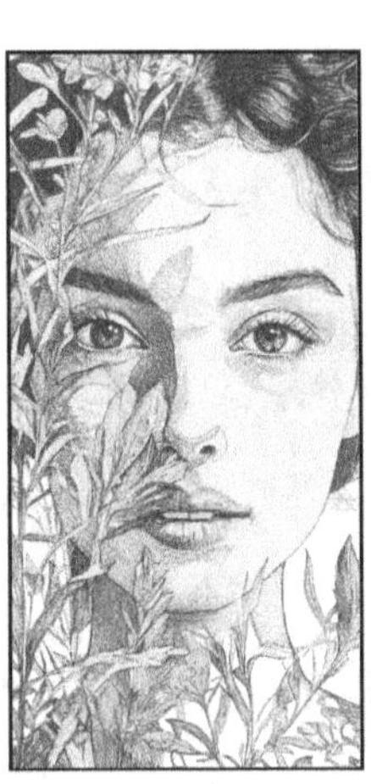
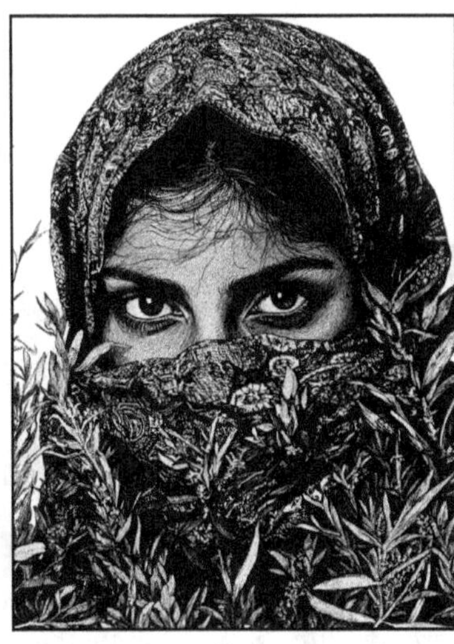
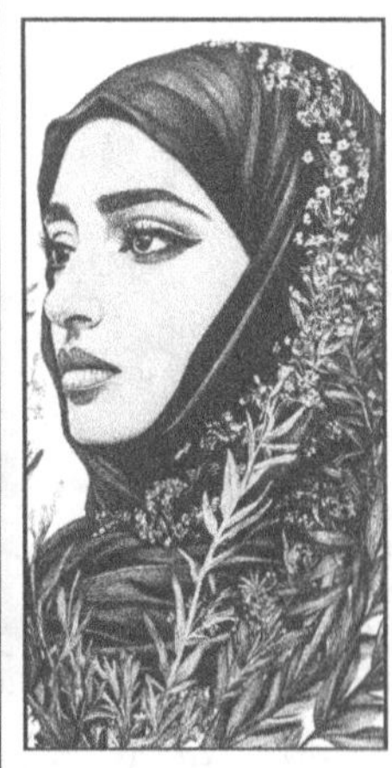

The desert, a vast expanse of sand and rock, stretches from the Levant to the edge of the Arabian Peninsula. In these landscapes where aridity reigns supreme and life seems to cling to each oasis, the Bedouin peoples have forged an intimate knowledge of their environment, developing ancestral knowledge adapted to these extreme conditions. Isolated by the vast desert landscapes, the women of these tribes have received and passed down healing and nurturing traditions based on resilient desert plants. This wisdom, born out of necessity and reverence for the natural world, showcases a centuries-old adjustment to the demands of an unforgiving environment.

Tattoos among Bedouin Women

In Bedouin communities, tattoos hold a profound significance in the female journey of transformation. These enduring symbols, etched onto the skin of women, serve as not just decorative embellishments but also as representations of safeguarding, abundance, and the shift into a fresh chapter of existence.

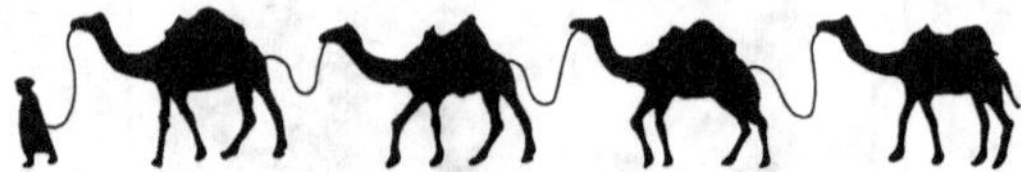

Tattooing amidst Bedouin women is frequently carried out utilizing black ink, created from soot, breast milk, or local plants like indigo. The patterns, typically geometric or symbolic, are administered to the face, hands, and occasionally other body parts, using a needle or thorn. This challenging procedure signifies a significant milestone, such as puberty or marriage, and is frequently accompanied by chants, prayers and devotions, fortifying the connection between the tangible and the divine.

In Bedouin culture, tattoos serve as a shield against negativity and harm. The symbols etched on the skin act as a barrier, safeguarding the woman's journey and prosperity.

Plants of the Desert

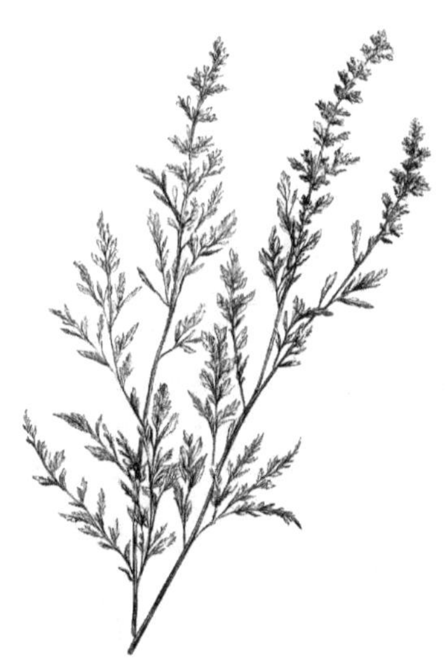

Mugwort (Artemisia herba-alba), known locally as **Shih**, holds significant value in Bedouin communities for its healing properties. It is utilized to alleviate menstrual discomfort, address digestive and respiratory issues, and for its antiseptic qualities. In traditions related to pregnancy and childbirth, mugwort is brewed to create herbal teas that offer comfort and support women during postnatal recovery.

Harmal (Peganum harmala) possesses potent healing and mystical qualities. The Bedouins harness its power to shield against malevolent forces and negative energy. Utilized in ceremonies, Harmal is ignited to cleanse the atmosphere and repel evil spirits, while its seeds are occasionally ingested as a remedy for menstrual discomfort. In the phases of childbirth, Harmal serves as a safeguard for both mother and child against detrimental energies.

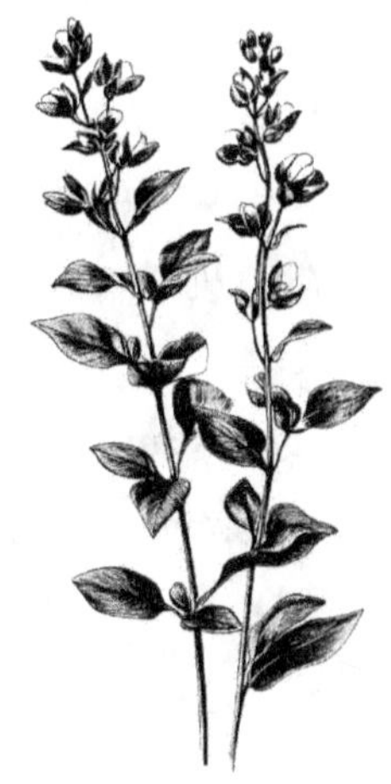

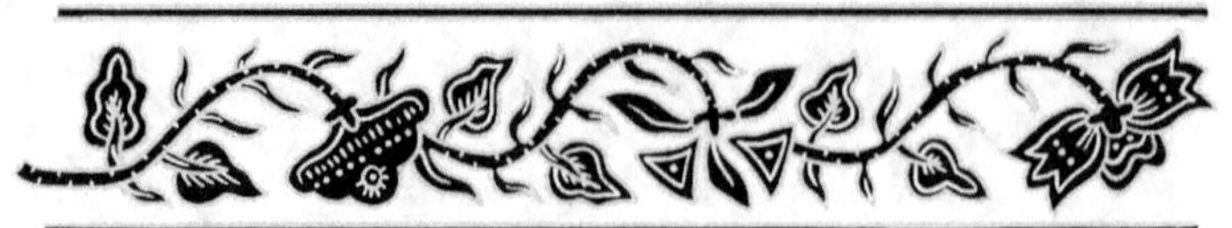

In every corner of the world, the secrets of women intertwined with plants thrive quietly, akin to hidden gardens within the depths of ancient traditions. Each woman, connected by a shared culture with her counterparts, holds within her a distinct wisdom, molded by her surroundings, her journey, and the subtle murmurs of her ancestors. These age-old customs, filled with taboos and subtlety, are frequently passed on in utmost confidentiality, shielded from external gazes, yet never entirely erased.

The traditional wisdom of women, encompassing health, body care, and intimate practices like natural contraception, persists, veiled within modernity. It remains subtle, nearly clandestine, yet far from stagnant; it transforms, adjusts, and withstands the demands of the present era. This wisdom, beyond a mere legacy, mirrors the strength of women, who, through every action, every remedy, sustain a profound bond with nature and the energies encircling them.

Even in this age of immediate knowledge and advancements in medicine, the wisdom of women endures, evolving gradually through interactions, creativity, and external influences, all the while safeguarding its core - a wisdom passed down discreetly from one generation to the next.

To Learn More

AFRICA

- Gueye, F. (2019). *The Healing Power of Senegal: Discovering the Medicinal Plants of Senegalese Tradition.* Pharmaceutical Sciences.
- *The West African Health Organization* (WAHO) published the West African Pharmacopoeia in 2013 in Ouagadougou.
- Bellakhdar, J. (1997). *Embracing Moroccan Heritage: Timeless Arab Healing and Community Wisdom.* Paris: Ibis Press.
- *Explore the captivating study on aromatic and medicinal plants in the Rif (Northern Morocco)* conducted by Chaachouay, N., Douira, A., Hassikou, R., Brhadda, N., & Dahmani, J. in 2020 at the Department of Biology - Ibn Tofail University - Kenitra.
- Fanny Colonna (2015). *Enchanting symbols and ceremonies of Kabyle women.* Editions La Découverte, Paris.
- Lemordant, D. (1969). *Enchanting and healing plants of the Fetishists of Oubangui (Bangui Region).* Journal of tropical agriculture and applied botany, 16(9), 3037. Persée.
- Neffati, M., Najja, H., & Matthew, Á. (Eds.) (2017). *Medicinal and Aromatic Plants of the World - Africa*, Volume 3. Springer, Dordrecht.
- Maoulida Mchangama and Pascale Salaün (2012). *Compiling a treasure trove in Mayotte.* Indian Ocean Studies, 48.

ASIA

- Kumar, S. & Yadav, S. (2013). *The Healing Power of India's Traditional Medicinal Plants: An Extensive Handbook.* New Delhi: Springer.
- Matilda Bupu Ria et al. (2021). *Enhancing the Impact: Ginger Warm Compress vs. Acidic Turmeric Consumption in Alleviating Primary Menstrual Pain Scale.* Journal of Maternal and Child Health.
- Kaptchuk, T. J. (2000). *The Web That Has No Weaver: Understanding Chinese Medicine.* Chicago: Contemporary Books.
- Takeda, S. (2015). *Embracing the Wisdom of Traditional Japanese Medicine: Kampo and the Healing Power of its Medicinal Plants.* Tokyo: Elsevier.

AMERICA

- Neihardt, J. G. (1932). *Black Elk Speaks: The Life Story of a Holy Man of the Oglala Sioux.* Lincoln: University of Nebraska Press.
- Brown, A. (2017). *Embracing Yoga: Nurturing and Transformation During the Menstrual Cycle.* London: HarperCollins.
- Avila, E., & Parker, J. (1999). *The Woman Who Glows in the Dark: A Curandera Reveals Traditional Aztec Secrets of Physical and Spiritual Health.* New York: Tarcher Perigee.
- Louise M. Burkhart's work on Healing practices in colonial Mexico published by the University of Arizona Press.
- Schultes, R. E., & Raffauf, R. F. (1990). *Embracing the Forest: Medicinal and Toxic Plants of the Northwest Amazonia.* Portland: Dioscorides Press.
- Irene Silverblatt's work *"Moon, Sun, and Witches: Gender Ideologies and Class in Inca and Colonial Peru"* published by Princeton University Press.
- Bilby, K. M., & Handler, J. S. (2012). *Manifesting Strength: The Criminalization of Obeah in the Anglophone Caribbean, 1760-2011.* University Press of the Caribbean.

OCEANIA

- Clarke, P. A. (2008). *Embracing the Wisdom of Aboriginal Plant Collectors: The Beautiful Connection Between Botanists and Australian Aboriginal People in the Nineteenth Century.*
- O'Neill, M., Soaki, I., & Tulo, S. (2014). *Healing Flora in Papua New Guinea. Papua New Guinea National Department of Health and the World Health Organization.*
- Best, E. (1924). *The Maori Division of Time.* Dominion Museum Bulletin.

GENERAL

- Mendlinger, S. (2020). Researcher's Reflection: Exploring Menstruation Throughout Time and Culture. In The Palgrave Handbook of Critical Menstruation Studies (pp. 441-447). Palgrave McMillan.
- Qasim, A. (2019, October 18). How people worldwide celebrate periods. ActionAid UK. Retrieved August 7, 2024.

EUROPE

- Ivanov, M. (2008). *Russian Folk Medicine: Ancient Wisdom of Eastern European Healing.* New York: Kensington Books.
- Festy, D. (2016). *My Guide to Essential Oils.* Leduc Publishing.
- Battaglia, S. (2003). *The Comprehensive Handbook of Aromatherapy.* Brisbane: The International Centre of Holistic Aromatherapy.
- Ellis, H. R. (1968). *The Path to Hel: An Exploration of the Perception of the Deceased in Ancient Norse Writings.* Cambridge: Cambridge University Press.

MIDDLE EAST

- Hanne Schönig, *The Body and Rites of Passage among Yemeni Women.* Reflecting on the Muslim Worlds and the Mediterranean, 113-114 | 2006, 167-177.
- Zargari, A. (1992). *Botanical Wonders of Iran.* Published by Tehran University Press.
- Bailey, C., & Danin, A. (1981). *Embracing the Magic of Bedouin Plant Utilization in Sinai and the Negev.* Economic Botany, 35(2), 145-162. Springer Nature.
- Ghazanfar, S. A. (1994). *Compendium of Arabian Medicinal Plants.* CRC Press.

A PRESENT
exclusive
AWAITS YOU.

• • •

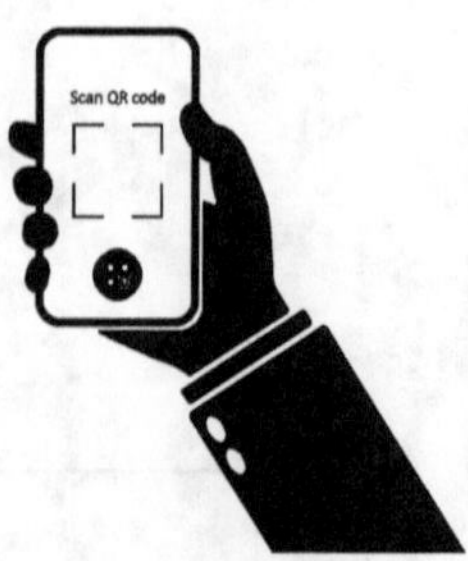

Shall we proceed with the
adventure?
Discover the magic within this
QR code!

Original title :
Relieve Menstrual Pain With Herbal Remedies
Ancestral Healing Knowledge of Women

© 2024, Vergers du Monde

Authored by Hélène Bourry, as a writer for Vergers du Monde.
Collection : World Agricultural Knowledge
Book Collection Number : 6

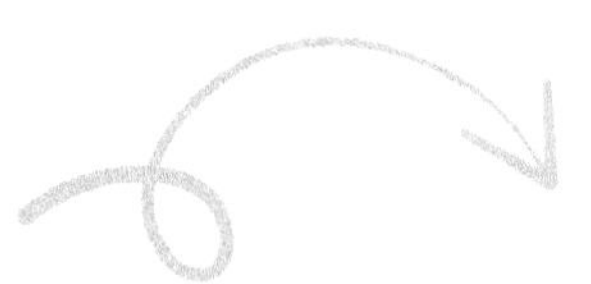

DON'T MISS OUR NEXT PRACTICAL GUIDES!

Join our newsletter for monthly agricultural insights.

VISIT US ONLINE

www.vergersdumonde.org

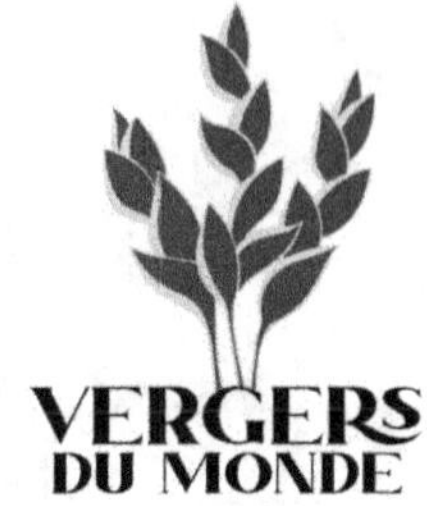

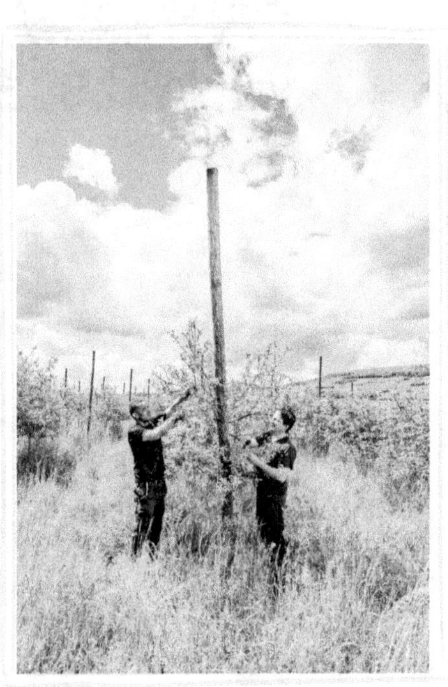

YOUR OPINION MATTERS TO US.

This book may have touched, inspired, or simply accompanied you for a moment, your feedback can truly make a difference.

Just a few words are enough to help other readers discover it, support our independent work, and show that these topics resonate.

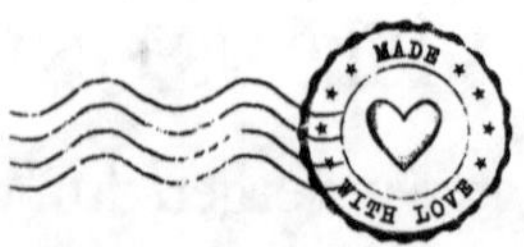